THE
MODEL
METHOD

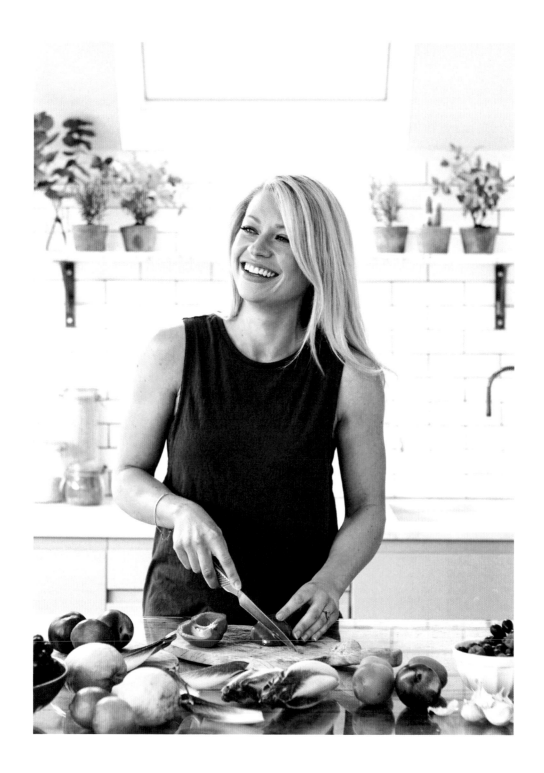

THE
MODEL
METHOD

Recipes, HIIT and Pilates exercises
for lifelong wellness

Hollie Grant

Owner of PilatesPT

piatkus

PIATKUS
First published in Great Britain in 2017 by Piatkus

1 3 5 7 9 10 8 6 4 2

A CIP catalogue record for this book
is available from the British Library.

ISBN 978-0-349-41613-7

Designed by Hart Studio
Recipe and cover photography by Nassima Rothacker
Fitness photography by Claire Pepper
Home economist and food styling by Natalie Thomson
Prop styling by Olivia Wardle
Clothing supplied by Sweaty Betty
Illustrations by Rodney Paull

Printed and bound in Germany by Mohn Media

Papers used by Piatkus are from well-managed forests and other responsible sources

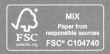

Piatkus
An imprint of
Little, Brown Book Group
Carmelite House
50 Victoria Embankment
London EC4Y 0DZ
An Hachette UK Company
www.hachette.co.uk
www.improvementzone.co.uk

Disclaimer
*The dietary information and exercises in this book are not intended to replace or conflict with the advice
given to you by your GP or other health professionals. All matters regarding your health should be discussed
with your GP. The author and publisher disclaim any liability directly or indirectly from the use of the material
in this book by any person.*

CONTENTS

6.   **INTRODUCTION**

14.   NOURISH

16.   Why diets are not the answer

18.   Government guidelines for a healthy lifestyle

30.   Obesity – the facts

32.   What is fat, then?

37.   Mindfulness – how a healthy mind creates a healthy body

40.   Eating seasonally

42.   Your nourish recipes

112.   STRENGTHEN

114.   What is Pilates?

118.   Anatomy 101

122.   Your muscle guide

128.   Common posture types

134.   Preventing muscle imbalances

135.   The Pilates principles and The Model Method

139.   Your strengthen exercises

182.   SWEAT

185.   What happens to our bodies when we exercise?

194.   What is HIIT?

198.   HIIT and The Model Method

201.   Your sweat exercises

248.   **CONCLUSION**

250.   **REFERENCES**

252.   **INDEX**

256.   **ACKNOWLEDGEMENTS**

INTRODUCTION

THE DIET MYTH

Fad diets. A Mars bar a day and ten cigarettes. Cabbage soup. Water mixed with maple syrup, cayenne and lemon. Ladies what are we doing to ourselves?! In the six years I have worked in the fitness industry, the 14 years I spent living with girlfriends and the 30 years I have been part of a world that chooses women's looks over their capabilities, I have heard of every diet under the sun. I've known of women who have eaten only fruit for two weeks. Who've suffered awful stomach cramps from wearing 'waist trainers' to bed. And, potentially the worst of all, women who have literally soiled themselves after taking diet pills. You may have attempted some of these types of diet yourself or know someone else who has, but don't worry – you are not alone and should in no way be ashamed! Dieting and fitness have become an increasingly large part of our culture and the media enjoy nothing more than reviewing the newest wellness trend or fad. My heart breaks every time I hear of a new aesthetic trend. We've had #thighgap, #bikinibridge and #abcrack. Looking through the social media photos from these trends, I see only women, no men.

So why is it that at any one time one in five of us in the UK is on a diet? [1] These diets obviously aren't working otherwise we would not be in a situation where 57 per cent of women in the UK are overweight or obese. [2] In fact, studies suggest that people on calorie-restricting diets can end up heavier than when they started. [3] It therefore seems reasonable to assume that some diets are ineffective and unhealthy, and some are incredibly dangerous. It could also be that these diets are so ridiculous that following them is all but impossible. Either way, something isn't working. Yet the number of diet and 'clean-eating' books being published shows no sign of slowing down. We still follow them, hoping that each new fad will be the diet that finally makes us happy. Spoiler alert: losing weight will not guarantee happiness. Being content with what you have and treating your body with kindness and gratitude will.

So let's take a look at exercise instead. If we were to believe all we saw in magazines and on social media, then we might think the number of women exercising is on the up. Simply search the hashtag for fitness inspiration (#fitspo) on Instagram and you'll be inundated with six packs and tight butts galore. However, the power of advertising strikes again. The reality is that only 10 per cent of adults in the UK play sport regularly and that 44 per cent do no moderate physical activity at all. [4] So almost half of us do nothing. We have access to free online fitness videos, more gyms than ever before and numerous government initiatives, yet we still choose to rest rather than sweat (or, even worse, diet instead of exercise).

It is so easy to feel compelled to change your eating habits or exercise choices based on what you see on social media when, in reality, we should make life choices for ourselves. We should choose our dinner based on what we would like to eat, not what looks good on Instagram. We should work out because we love how it makes us feel, not because a magazine says that Jennifer Aniston does it for three hours a day, every day (this is a complete guess). The sad thing is that seeing all these fit, beautiful women on social media is quite possibly having an adverse effect on our fitness motivation, especially when so many of them are airbrushed. Modern-day advertising means that we see more of other women's bodies than our own at times – and, if we don't see the reality of exercise (sweaty red faces, frizzy scraped-back topknots, wedgies, crotch sweat patches and bodies of all shapes and sizes) then we are always going to feel like we are abnormal. Worse still, we may feel everyone else is thinking we're abnormal too. A study by Sport England found that 75 per cent of the women they surveyed wanted to take part in sport but felt held back for fear of being judged on their appearance and ability [5] – what an amazing waste of talent. The irony is that regular exercise would improve our ability and potentially make us care less about our appearance. Chances are we are all so worried about our own ability we aren't even noticing anyone else's.

So, despite the swathes of avocados, skimpy leggings and head-standing yogis, it appears we are not yet all aboard the wellness wagon. We need to remember that social media, for many, is a business. The photos posted are often chosen to promote the account holder's product, services or personality. They are not a true reflection of real life and they are providing little education to us on our bodies, how they move and how most of us should really be eating. I hope this book will give you more insight into your body and health than any scrolling through social media ever could.

Worryingly, it's not just adults who are struggling to prioritise exercise in their lives; this problem is rubbing off on our children too. Around 40 per cent of 16-year-old girls take part in no vigorous physical activity at all.[5] And this is at an age when children have more free time than they will ever have as adults. A study carried out by Girlguiding in 2016 found that fear of people criticising their body stops 41 per cent of girls aged between 11 and 16 from taking part in exercise, whilst 51 per cent of them felt they should lose weight. Moreover, only 61 per cent of them are happy with how they look – how incredibly sad that, at an age when girls should be free from the constraints of body shaming and pressure to look a certain way, so few of them feel this way.[6]

All this data points to the possibility that, despite knowing more than we've ever known about the importance of eating well and exercising, we are simply not managing to do so. This needs to change!

ABOUT ME

Nine years ago I graduated from my psychology degree, full of excitement and hope, and set off in a completely different direction to start my dream apprenticeship as a chocolatier in London. I had planned on a career in chocolate since I was young and I had secured a degree just in case it didn't work out, meanwhile travelling to London to carry out work experience with my eventual employer. A year after taking on my dream apprenticeship, I was underweight, overworked and suffering with depression. I'd spent a whole year forcing myself to stick with the role because it was all I'd ever wanted to do and was a great opportunity, but my health and happiness were really suffering and life is just too short. One day I woke up and my exhausted body made the decision for me that I would never step into a commercial kitchen again.

As they say, everything happens for a reason, and I took a role as a receptionist in a Pilates studio while I decided what to do next. I had always been heavily involved in sport growing up: I was a 100 metre sprinter during my years in a military boarding school and had a father who was in the Parachute Regiment (I think I inherited my competitiveness from him). However, though I had decided the military wasn't for me, I had never considered a career in fitness. Thinking back, I had witnessed so many friends suffer with disordered eating over the years – my university dissertation was even on 'eating disorders in first-year students' – but I had just never made the link to the possibility of helping others to feel at ease with their bodies.

I quickly realised how much my lack of exercise over the past year had affected my mental health. The catering industry works such long hours, plus it's a physically demanding job, and I had managed to do no exercise for a year. As soon as I started working in the Pilates studio, I fell in love with the method. Pilates seemed to be all about making your body strong, flexible, functional and comfortable. It was not about being skinny or losing weight. I loved how it made my body feel and it held my interest like no other technique before. I quickly became studio manager before being motivated by my instructors to take the STOTT Pilates training course to become a Pilates instructor myself, and later completed my personal trainer qualifications.

After teaching thousands of classes, I was even more certain that Pilates was incredible (I'd used it to prepare for my eight marathons in eight days charity event). But there was something missing. My clients enjoyed their sessions and were incredibly strong, with beautiful posture, but their cardiovascular fitness was lacking. If you love a certain form of exercise, it's easy to put all your eggs in one basket. My clients would often say that they hated running/spinning/swimming so just didn't bother doing it, but this didn't sit well with me. I then discovered the world of high-intensity interval training (HIIT). All the research into HIIT seemed too good to be true. You only had to do short, tough bursts of exercise? And it was more effective than long periods of cardiovascular endurance training? It couldn't be true – but the science backs it up. I began adding short periods of HIIT into my private clients' Pilates practice and the results were incredibly positive. Their endurance, strength, functionality and self-confidence all improved, plus those who had high (and health-damaging) levels of body fat found those levels decreased. My clients felt empowered watching what their bodies could do and how strong they were becoming. It felt as if HIIT and Pilates were the perfect combination, and much like a model pupil this was the model method. The Model Method was born.

Three years ago, I set up my own studio – PilatesPT. I wanted a private studio that clients could chat in, train in, cry in and feel supported in by female instructors – somewhere totally unintimidating. A studio that would improve women's confidence, not dent it, and that would teach women that what their bodies can do is more important than what they look like. This is exactly what our studio and The Model Method have become known for. I also wanted to afford my training and message to everyone, not just those who trained with me in the studio. I therefore created The Model Method Online, which offers the same exercises, advice and support that I provide to all of my clients. I hope this book will help you discover your healthiest, strongest, happiest body too and rid you of any self-doubt, poor body image and negative body goals.

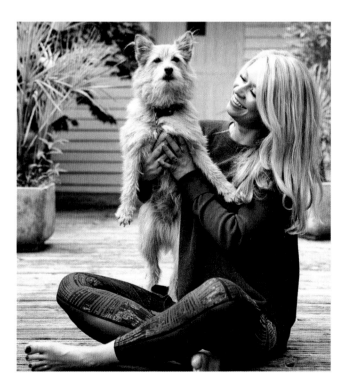

WHY IS THIS BOOK DIFFERENT?

As someone who works in the fitness industry, my aim is, and has always been, to motivate women to exercise to be strong and healthy, and live long, fulfilling lives – not to look a certain way. I do not believe in aggressive exercising. I do not believe in diets. I don't even believe that *all* exercise is good for you. I believe that we should exercise as and when we can, because we enjoy it and want to do it. I don't want women to exercise because they have eaten too much over Christmas or have a holiday coming up. When we exercise for these reasons, it's because we feel we are not good enough as we are. We believe our bodies won't look good enough in a bikini, or we have lost control over the festive period and believe we must fix this. We are assigning negativity to exercise and over the years this leads to the feeling that exercise is to be dreaded, like getting a bikini wax. If instead we see exercise as something positive because we know we will feel great afterwards, because it reduces our risk of life-threatening illnesses and because it will give us more energy, then there is no reason it can't be as appealing as going for a facial. It is all about how we view exercise, and unfortunately years of false advertising and supposedly quick-fix diets have made us lose sight of what exercise is truly about.

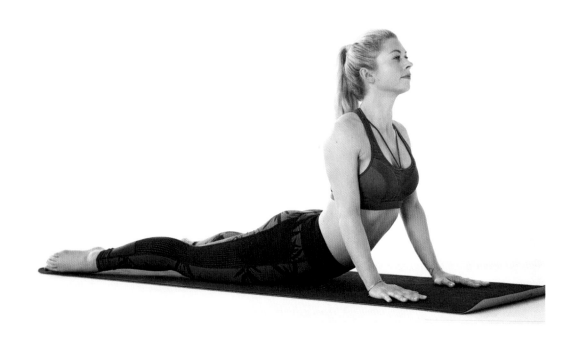

This book is not a diet plan. It is not going to tell you the secrets of weight loss because there are none. It's not really even going to tell you what you should and shouldn't eat. It is, however, going to give you the insight into what exercise and food does to our bodies so you can take ownership of your health. I have spent the past six years trying to spread the message that learning to love exercise, and to love the food you eat, is the key to lifelong wellness. There are no quick fixes (and there need be none if exercise is simply part of your life). Health has no time frame. It's a long-term journey that needn't involve abstention or pain. I really hope this book inspires you to give exercise another go, or try something new, and see exercise in a more positive, appealing light.

HOW TO USE THE MODEL METHOD

As more and more of my clients felt the benefits of The Model Method, I realised I wanted everyone to have access to it, anytime, anywhere. I loved the thought of women around the world putting 30 minutes a day aside to move their bodies in a safe, empowering and positive way. I therefore created The Model Method Online – a personalised online version of our in-studio training. This involves 30-minute HIIT and 15-minute Pilates workouts. It is all about sweating with HIIT, strengthening with Pilates and nourishing your body with food you enjoy creating as much as you enjoy eating it. Now, by putting my experience, knowledge and recipes into this book, I hope that even more women around the world can start improving their health and happiness.

The book is split into three chapters: Nourish, Strengthen and Sweat. These chapters cover the areas of wellness I believe truly contribute to a healthy, strong body. The Nourish section will re-educate you on the main food groups and on how they contribute to your health and wellness, and I'll help you to address the topic of mindful eating. The recipes included in this section are for inspiration – this is not a diet plan! I believe that food is to be enjoyed, not restricted. I feel that, if we take time over the preparation, the cooking and the eventual eating of our food, we reduce our risk of binge and emotional eating. The more stress and negativity we put around our diet, the more we lose sight of when we are truly hungry; we must learn to listen to the feedback our body is giving us. The recipes are a collection of some of my favourite meals. My experience as a chef taught me to really pay attention to the taste, smell and feel of my ingredients, and food is an important part of my life. The collection includes all food groups, but if you are vegan, vegetarian or have any intolerances, each recipe has replacements and recommendations.

You may be wondering what qualifications I have to advise you on what to eat. This is where the incredible, inspirational registered nutritionist Laura Thomas, PhD. comes in. When I decided to write this book, I wanted to ensure I wasn't going to add to the swathes of pseudoscience out there. I didn't want to confuse people even more or give misleading advice. Laura is a straight-talking, no-bullshit, science-loving nutritionist. You can find out all about the amazing, super-talented career she has forged at laurathomasphd.co.uk (seriously, check her out!).

Once I had written up my favourite recipes, I passed them on to Laura for her expert opinion and asked her to give me her nutritional advice on them. Her response was inspiring. When she sent back her report, I could see that some of the recipes were a little high in fat whereas some were a little low in fat. Some could have more carbohydrates in, some could have less. I was so disappointed, borderline heartbroken (I know that sounds extreme but I'd poured my heart into the recipes). I asked Laura if I should go back and change them to make them more 'textbook healthy' and she told me this (in her no-bullshit way): 'Well you could, but that'd be crazy. If these are the recipes you love, and they taste delicious, and you're not saying eat this carbonara every meal, then why would you change them? Balance is important and not every meal has to be nutritionally "perfect". The whole point is to teach people to eat food they enjoy and move more and not obsess over counting calories.' (I told you she's awesome.) And Laura is right.

I am not an endorser of diets that remove whole food groups. Nor am I interested in telling you to cut out carbs (how the hell would your body have the energy to exercise without carbs?). What I do want you to do is learn to love food again. To learn to enjoy shopping for delicious, quality ingredients that were grown or made with love. I want you to have a think about what you would like for dinner and then make it yourself. Food that you have made, with passion and attention, is infinitely more satisfying than a ready meal, and it'll most likely have far less crap in it too! Anyway, I digress . . .

Your Strengthen chapter is all about Pilates! Here we will discuss the history of Joseph Pilates (yes, Pilates was an actual person) and the benefits to your body. You will learn how the body moves and functions, and what muscle imbalances are. Using this information, you can assess your own posture and decide which Pilates exercises you would like to use first. Your Pilates exercises will be broken down into areas – the lower body, the core and the upper body. Each exercise will have a clear description of what type of posture it will benefit, the muscles it works and how to make it easier or harder as your strength improves. You will need no equipment, other than a yoga mat, and you will be practising your Pilates exercises every other day (three days per week) for 15 minutes. Those who practise Pilates often find that they consider their posture more in day-to-day life, and that they suffer fewer aches and pains.

Finally, you have your Sweat chapter. This is all about High Intensity Interval Training, or HIIT. You'll learn all about how your body's energy systems work and why HIIT has a multitude of health benefits. I'll explain the science behind HIIT and how best to practise it. I have split your HIIT exercises into the same three groups: exercises for the lower body, the core and then the upper body. Again, you will only need a yoga mat and will practise your sweat exercises every other day – three days per week – for between 18 and 30 minutes, depending on your fitness levels. Once you have read this book and have created a picture of your current strengths and weaknesses, you can choose which areas you'd like to work on first. Each exercise will be explained in depth, and I will show you which muscles it will target and how to adapt the exercise to suit you.

As a rule of thumb, I like my clients to wait 48 hours between HIIT workouts to allow their glycogen levels to replenish. You will alternate your workouts between the sweat and strengthen exercises each day, with one rest day each week. A week of The Model Method could therefore look like this:

Monday	Sweat workout
Tuesday	Strengthen workout
Wednesday	Sweat workout
Thursday	Strengthen workout
Friday	Sweat workout
Saturday	Strengthen workout
Sunday	Rest day

Remember that The Model Method is designed to improve your health, strength and happiness, so please do not beat yourself up if you miss some workouts. This is about a lifestyle change, not a quick fix. Moving a little, every day, is one of the best feelings, so let's make sure exercise is a positive addition to your life! Enjoy it, savour it and use it as an opportunity to be mindful of your body's capabilities. This is the beginning of an amazing journey and I can't wait for you to get started.

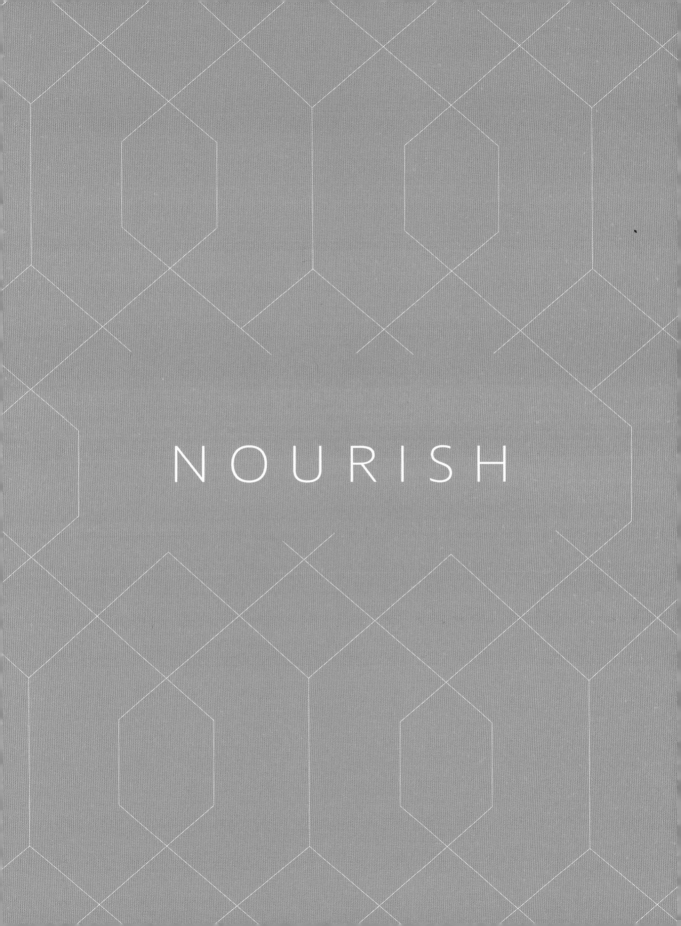

NOURISH

NOURISH

It's not the size that counts, it's what you do with it that matters. Yes, I've lowered the tone – but I'm talking about our bodies, of course. Increasingly, research shows that health is not necessarily determined by our size; it's what we're doing with our bodies that counts. Over the years, we've been taught that the bigger the dress size, the less healthy we are. We are subjected to a fat-shaming culture that teaches us that only those who are slim, flexible and glowing are healthy, and if we don't fit this ideal we are unwell, lazy and weak. But this really isn't accurate. Not when being 'overweight' doesn't necessarily correlate with poor health. Not when our body shapes and sizes have a lot to do with genetics. Not when different types of fat mean different things, and not all fat can be seen. If we can't see what's going on inside our bodies, how on earth can we judge ourselves on the way we look? It is a hypocritical world that judges people so aggressively on the size of their clothes while 19 per cent of the UK still smoke (smoking is still the largest single preventable cause of cancer in the UK). [7] We need to take our focus away from what we weigh and focus more on what we do to our bodies if we really want lifelong wellness.

A study involving 334,164 European men and women found that increasing your physical activity, no matter your body mass index (BMI) or waist circumference, reduced your risk of death. Over the 12-year monitoring period, the researchers found that physical inactivity resulted in twice as many deaths as a high BMI (over 30). This is a gentle reminder to move more, not necessarily diet more, if you want to reduce your risk of death. We presume that our weight defines our health, but our behaviours can have a greater influence. [8]

WHY DIETS ARE NOT THE ANSWER TO HEALTH, HAPPINESS OR WEIGHT LOSS

In the media, and even in the health sector, overweight people are described as a 'burden on the economy'. Negativity towards those who are overweight is often hidden under the guise of caring about someone's health. The same amount of pressure, however, is not put on those who don't eat fruit and vegetables. Or those who don't get enough sleep. Or those with poor stress-management skills (these are all issues that can have a negative effect on your health). With this increasing pressure and emphasis on weight rather than health, it's no wonder we are all reaching for the next diet plan. Let's take a look at what those diets are doing to our bodies.

OK, so we've decided we want to lose weight (mistake number one) and asked our friend Beth how she lost that 6 kilograms for her wedding last year (which by now she has put back on plus a bit more, because that's what diets have been shown to do to you). She tells you she ate less/ate only protein/ate only fruit/did a juice cleanse/ate only baby food/took diet pills with only the best intentions of improving her health. So you pick a day to start (probably a Monday as we all like a 'clean start') and decide that you'll have one last blowout/treat yourself to a night on the town/eat all the chocolate left in the house/order a takeaway at the weekend as a final treat before the diet begins. Monday comes and you're excited to get started. You've spent a fortune on a juicer/organic meat/baby food but it's worth it, right? By Wednesday all you can think about is cake. By Thursday you've pissed off your whole family and cried in front of your boss. By Saturday you've had a 'fuck it' moment and eaten a whole jar of Nutella all ready to start the same cycle again on Monday.

Sound familiar? Of course it does. We've all been there (if you haven't you'll know someone who has) and it is absolutely no reflection on your levels of willpower. It does not make you weak. It makes you human. How the hell do you expect your body to not fight back? Your body is freaking clever.

When we embark on an eating plan that doesn't support our energy demands or metabolism, our body is well equipped to disagree. Our bodies are amazing at making sure things stay in equilibrium and that we don't starve ourselves (your body needs the calories you are depriving it of in order to function). Our bodies have many tricks up their sleeves to prevent you completing crazy diets, and these tricks are far more powerful than anyone's willpower.

Take skipping lunch, for example. You're under the misguided assumption that it'll help you lose weight. When our bodies realise we have forgotten lunch, they say, 'hold on, everyone, she's forgotten to eat. Can everyone just hold on tight to what they've got, maybe slow down your work for the day, just in case she doesn't manage to get any food until later?' So the effect is you feel sluggish, and your body reserves all its energy (i.e. your metabolism slows down).

Then you manage to make it to dinner without food, but by now your body has been saying, 'OK guys, let's give her more ghrelin (the hormone that tells you you're hungry) so she puts finding food on her priority list'. Your body thinks it's helping you out. It's reminding you to feed it. So, by the time you do have dinner, you have a hunger like no other. You'll feel like you want to eat your dinner *and* the lunch you missed. The potential for bingeing is high.

Being on a diet requires you to think about every decision you make about food like you're choosing the next prime minister. You're counting calories/macros/which cake you'd eat first as if you were on death row. When your mind is so focused on food, plus your body is on a go-slow because you are eating less, it's impossible to stay as focused on your job, relationships or health. Chances are you'll have little energy to exercise (which is the real hero here) and your mood will be affected.

You will be ignoring your body's natural hunger signals, and these are incredibly important and powerful feedback mechanisms.

Don't do it.

Studies suggest that diets have negative long-term effects not only on your health but also on your relationship with food. Growing evidence suggests that those who try to achieve and maintain a weight-suppressed state are at risk of a binge-eating disorder and there is literature connecting yo-yo dieting with compromised health, including increased mortality and some forms of cancer. To put it bluntly, those who diet the most have a higher death rate than non-dieters. [9]

Food is to be enjoyed, tasted, prepared, smelt, shared and loved. It is fuel for the body, nourishment for the soul and most importantly essential. We have to eat, so why not make it a positive experience? You will soon see that once we take the negativity out of food, we make more positive health choices.

WHAT ARE THE GOVERNMENT GUIDELINES FOR A 'HEALTHY LIFESTYLE'?

Now I know it's not always sexy, or exciting, to follow government guidelines. We all want to follow what the beautiful young model tells us to do so we can look like her. But remember that the government bodies responsible for these guidelines have a huge team of scientists, advisers and academics consulting with each other to come up with the safest, most thoroughly researched advice on what we as a population should eat. Now remember these are just that – guidelines – and there is room for you to adapt them slightly if, say, you are vegetarian or lactose intolerant. For example, the starch foods guideline includes bread, but you may find bread doesn't sit right with you and therefore you might choose alternatives. Again, there are no big claims, no sweeping statements in government guidelines. However, they really are based on years of research and statistics, and have the best intentions – the government wants you to be healthy and free from disease, they are not trying to get you to buy into their 'brand'.

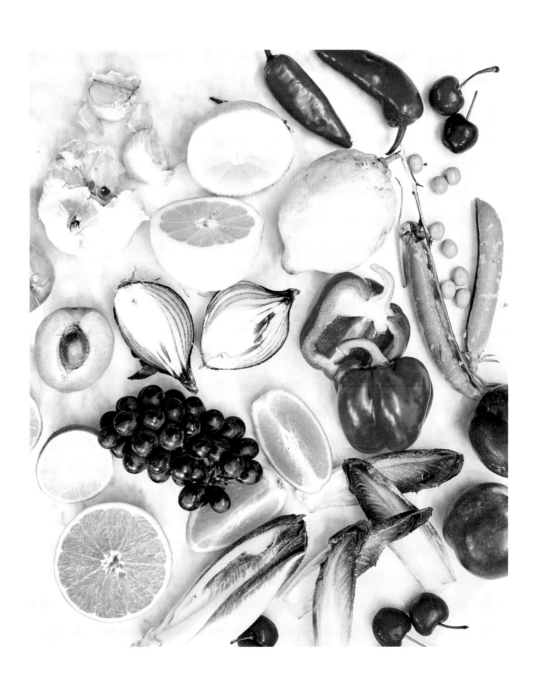

So let's take a look at each of these guidelines while delving into exactly what each food group is. These guidelines are taken from the Eatwell Guide, which was devised by the Food Standards Agency. [10]

EAT PLENTY OF VEGETABLES (AND SOME FRUIT)

Not only is this the guideline I'm listing first but I also honestly feel that this is the guideline we need to read, re-read and then write on a post-it note on our fridge door!

It is recommended that we eat at least five portions of fruit and/or vegetables per day. Around only three in ten adults in the UK actually manage this. [11] It's safe to say that we can all work on adding a little more in, especially when we consider that people whose diets are high in vegetables have a reduced risk of death and are less likely to develop cardiovascular disease. [12] And please remember the two words 'at least'. Don't be held back by this number! In Japan, the government guidelines are 13 portions of vegetables and four of fruit! The UK government is realistic in its recommendations (especially as 70 per cent of us don't even eat five a day) but really it could be higher. My favourite vegetable-rich recipes in this book are the Nourish Bowl (page 62) and Corn and Lime Fritters (page 50).

Most vegetables and fruits are low in fat, contain no cholesterol and are high in fibre (which, by the way, makes us poo – which is fantastic). They are an important source of vital nutrients that benefit every cell in the body and contain various vitamins and minerals. They are rich sources of potassium, folate and vitamin C, amongst many other micronutrients. Folate helps in the formation of red blood cells, vitamin A helps to protect the body against infections and vitamin C helps to heal wounds and cuts and aids iron absorption. It is thought that potassium can have an effect on lowering blood pressure.

Aim to base your meals around a variety of vegetables, of various colours. The colour of a vegetable can tell you a lot about the types of phytochemicals (compounds that benefit our health in various ways) inside it, so ensure you eat the rainbow and try not to just stick to your favourite five every day of the week. For example, red fruits and vegetables contain lycopene, which is a powerful antioxidant thought to reduce the risk of cancer (canned tomatoes have more than fresh ones, so don't underestimate canned veggies). Orange foods contain beta-carotene, which is converted to vitamin A by the body and helps to maintain healthy eyes. Get it. Eat them all. Eating fruit and vegetables with their skins on (except the obvious ones, such as bananas) adds an extra dose of fibre to your diet. Fibre is key to regular bowel movement and a happy gut – and most of us aren't getting enough!

Unfortunately, statistics show that the lowest earners eat the least vegetables. [11] If the limiting factor for you eating vegetables is their cost, try eating seasonally. It can cost a great deal more to buy a mango that has been grown in India and flown across the world to your supermarket than it does to buy some raspberries that were grown down the road. You'll also be helping to sustain local producers, eating far fresher (and hence more nutritious) food, and eating with the seasons as our ancestors would have done. You can read more about when your favourite fruit and vegetables are in season on page 41. Don't forget that canned and frozen vegetables are also valuable! Frozen vegetables are usually picked and frozen when at their best and their nutrients are locked in. They are a great addition to your freezer!

There are many ways of sneaking extra vegetables into your diet. Try adding grated courgette, carrot or celery to stews and casseroles to bulk out meals and add flavour. Create your own coleslaw with grated carrot, cabbage and onion and add apple cider vinegar and lemon juice rather than mayonnaise. Add dried figs or apricots to your porridge in the morning or add bananas to your muesli. Throw fruit and vegetables in at every possible meal and you can't go wrong!

BASE MEALS ON POTATOES, RICE, PASTA AND OTHER STARCHY CARBOHYDRATES

Most of us are already hitting this quota with the increasing quantities of long-life breads and white starchy foods in our diets. However, again, it's the types of starchy foods we are choosing that's important for our health. Starchy foods are a great source of energy and fibre and are our main source of carbohydrate. As well as starch, they contain iron and B vitamins. There have been many 'low-carb' diets out there and carbs seem to be feared by many. The phrase 'no carbs before Marbs' (shakes head) and the wrong belief that carbohydrates 'make you fat' have given this vital food group a bad name. *Any* food group that is consumed in high volumes and not used in the body is stored as fat. Plus carbohydrates only have half the energy value (in calories) of fat. Carbohydrates are vital, and are valuable for those planning on being more active. I absolutely love my Squash and Rosemary Carbonara (page 83) and Speltsotto (page 74) for dinner, especially if I have a long run planned for the following day (eating carbohydrate-rich foods before a long-distance run or cycle helps to ensure the muscles are full of usable energy). The Cashew and Oat Pancakes (page 84) are a great way to start a busy day.

When we eat carbohydrates, the body breaks them down into smaller sugars (glucose, galactose and fructose), which are absorbed by the body and used for energy. Glucose that isn't needed straight away is converted into glycogen and stored in the muscles and liver for later. These glycogen stores are not infinite and so, when the stores are full, the excess glucose is stored as fat. Glycogen is a great, readily available source of energy for exercise. It is needed for short, sharp bursts of exercise (such as HIIT) and is used during the first portion of any sport. Longer periods of less intense exercise can tap into fat reserves (carbohydrates are also used in this process). However, when the body hasn't got enough carbohydrate, it can start to eat into its protein stores. Protein is needed for growth and repair of muscles and, hence, if we do not have enough carbohydrate ready for use, we can hinder our body's ability to build new muscle (and hence improve our strength). This can be seen in long-distance runners, who can be very lean and have limited amounts of muscle. Their muscles are broken down to further fuel the body due to their intense energy requirements. This is not recommended and can put a great deal of stress on the body.

You'll often hear carbohydrates discussed in terms of whether they are 'simple' or 'complex'. By the end of the digestion process, they are essentially the same by-product (sugar), but the main difference is the time taken for each source of carbohydrate to be broken down into energy by the body. Simple sugars are quickly and easily broken down by the body and have a very immediate effect on blood-sugar levels. Simple sugars do have their place – for example, when athletes need a quick burst of energy for sport. For the rest of us, simple sugars are just a recipe for a rollercoaster rush followed by a rollercoaster plummet of emotions and energy – the kind we've all experienced post-chocolate bar. Simple sugars are typically found in foods that are sweet, such as soda, chocolate, candy and table sugar. If it helps, when you look at the amount of sugar listed on a product, eight grams is the equivalent of two teaspoons of sugar.

Complex sugars take longer to break down into their individual sugars and therefore leave us feeling fuller for longer and do not have the same erratic effect on our blood-sugar levels. They are also often high in fibre, which we know helps to promote healthy bowel movements. Examples are starchy vegetables (such as potatoes, sweet potatoes and squash) and wholegrains (such as oats, barley and rice).

When deciding which starches to include, try to keep them as close to what nature intended as possible. If we look at bread, for example, generally it counts as a starchy food, but some heavily processed forms (e.g. white long-life breads) can have high levels of sugar too. Also, the process of bleaching flour to create white bread can strip the wheat of some of its nutrients, although some companies now fortify their bread with calcium and iron so it's worth checking their ingredients lists. We should also consider the preservatives used to make sure the bread doesn't go mouldy too quickly. Don't get me wrong, sometimes there's nothing better than a slice of white toast with lashings of butter, but don't rely on that for your starch count as there are far better, more nutritious sources.

If you love bread, switch it up for wholegrain versions. Breads that are sourced directly from local bakers or made by you tend to have fewer preservatives as they are not expected to last as long. You can up your healthy starch count by roasting celeriac or squash wedges with garlic and rosemary instead of chips. You can substitute quinoa (delicious cooked in stock), barley or spelt in place of your usual rice or pasta dishes (as in my Speltsotto – see page 74) or add oats to pancake mixtures, cakes and even savoury dishes (a handful of oats in your lasagne mince will pad it out and barely be noticed). Baked white or sweet potatoes with their skins on are a simple lunch to take to work, and adding some oily fish such as mackerel or sardines is a real winner.

EAT DAIRY OR DAIRY ALTERNATIVES

Dairy is a great source of protein and calcium, both of which are important for bone health. Dairy has become a contentious topic over the past few years, with increasing numbers of people choosing to omit it from their diet. Many believe that dairy has a negative effect on their health or that they may have an intolerance to lactose (a sugar found in dairy products).

When we consume lactose, the enzyme lactase breaks the lactose into the sugars glucose and galactose. These sugars are easily absorbed into the bloodstream. Those with lactose intolerance don't produce enough lactase (if any), so lactose stays in their digestive system, where it's fermented by bacteria. This leads to the production of various gases (not ideal), which cause the symptoms associated with lactose intolerance. The main symptoms are wind, diarrhoea and a bloated stomach, which tend to present themselves within a few hours. Lactose intolerance is different to a dairy allergy, whereby the sufferer experiences an immune reaction with symptoms such as wheezing or a rash.

If you are worried you have a lactose intolerance, it's important to speak to your GP before cutting out a whole food group. There are many vegan sources of calcium but it isn't as simple as cutting out dairy and carrying on with your life – you would need to ensure you were substituting calcium with greens such as kale, collard greens and broccoli. If you are choosing to drink dairy alternatives, try to choose those that are fortified and unsweetened.

Some people also worry about the high levels of antibiotics that modern-day cattle are fed to prevent them from getting ill. As with all animal products, what the animal eats is ultimately transferred to you (but in varying doses). If this worries you, seek out organic products, which, while more expensive, are becoming more common in supermarkets. In general, organic products (in the case of beef) will be derived from cattle that have been allowed to graze, that have not been treated with most drugs and that have been fed on organically certified feed. They also have the highest animal welfare standards – keeping cows indoors their whole life is banned under organic standards. Due to their very nature, organic products are more expensive and, while it would be lovely to purchase only organic dairy, this just may not be possible for many of us. I started by swapping the milk I drank to organic. Small changes all add up, but do not feel any pressure to go organic if it is not a concern for you.

So, those of you who do eat dairy, hello. Cheese, as insanely delicious as it is, should not be a *large* part of your diet. While the amount varies from cheese to cheese, specific types can have high levels of saturated fat (if you're looking for a lower fat variety, mozzarella is an example of a nice compromise as it's low fat but still delicious). Where possible, eat cheese in small amounts (Parmesan has a strong taste so not much is needed) and try to aim for lower fat cheeses where possible. Aim to use semi-skimmed milk, don't include too much cream in your diet, and cook with butter for flavour by all means but use oils such as olive or rapeseed where possible.

My Sunday ritual for a long time has been cheese and crackers for lunch. I love slabs of Comté on a fig cracker with caramelised onion chutney. It's delicious and I enjoy this tradition more than most, but I'm not doing it every day. I don't really eat any cheese during the week. We must remember that these are guidelines for how to eat the majority of the time; don't feel under pressure to cut out all of your treats and traditions. Everything in moderation – and because you want it, not need it. That's why the Chocolatier's Hot Chocolate on page 101 is my favourite dairy fix!

EAT BEANS, PULSES, FISH, EGGS, MEAT AND OTHER NON-DAIRY SOURCES OF PROTEIN

Protein is needed for growth and development and is an important component of every cell in the body. We use protein to create enzymes, hormones and other body chemicals. We also use it to build new muscle and repair it after exercise. Proteins are made of small compounds called amino acids, which are the building blocks of the body. There are 22 different amino acids and the body can make all but nine of them (these nine are called 'essential amino acids' as we can only get them through eating them). Different foods have different amino acids in, so if we were to only eat one type of food all day (I'd choose chocolate) we probably wouldn't have eaten all of the amino acids we need. This is why we need to ensure we eat a balanced diet. The Baked Black Beans (page 46) are an amazing source of protein, especially if you opt for the poached egg too, and the Steak and Black Bean Burritos (page 80) are absolutely delicious.

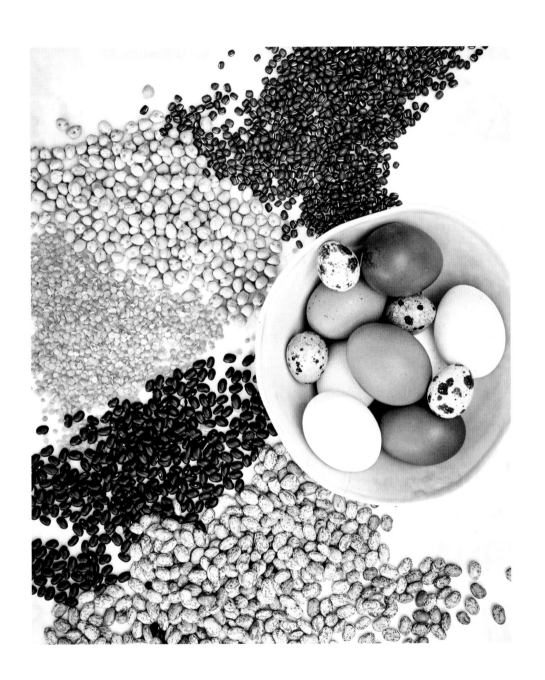

Animal proteins such as meat and eggs contain all of our essential amino acids, making them 'complete proteins'. If we choose not to eat animal products, as vegans do, we have to be mindful of finding a way to eat all of these essential amino acids. For example, quinoa and soy beans are complete proteins. Pulses, beans, lentils, tofu and hemp are good sources of protein and are great for adding fibre to your diet (I'm all about those regular bowel movements!).

Protein's main job is to build or repair muscle, and this is why we are used to those who do a lot of exercise (particularly body builders) discussing protein shakes – they wish to supplement their protein intake to allow muscle growth. Actual increase in the size of a muscle mostly only happens in males – women do not have high enough levels of testosterone for this to happen easily. If you're wondering how female bodybuilders manage this, they spend years and years, hours upon hours, with often the most advanced training techniques creating the incredible bodies they have. If you eat a few eggs and lift a few times a week, it will not make you a female bodybuilder. I mentioned earlier that, during exercise, if our carbohydrate levels are too low, we can end up breaking down the proteins in our muscles for use as energy. Well, protein is also used to repair muscles after exercise. When we exercise, we make tiny tears in our muscles (don't worry, it's a good thing) and this is what we can feel usually about 48 hours later. If you've ever felt that deep ache in your muscles where it's hard to get up off the loo or lift up your child, chances are you have suffered from DOMS (delayed-onset muscle soreness). The reason many people choose to take protein shakes after exercise is that protein can help with the recovery of those tiny tears. It has been recommended that eating said protein soon after your workout is beneficial and so a small pot of (sugar-free) yoghurt or an egg could help.

If you do choose to drink protein shakes, please be careful which ones you choose. Protein powders can taste disgusting and so some companies are adding sugars and sweeteners to them to make them more palatable (there's even a cookie-dough-flavoured one). Do you really want to be pumping all those additives into your body when you could so easily eat something that's far closer to what nature intended. Personally, I give protein shakes a wide berth unless I recognise the ingredients.

Aim to spread your protein intake out across the day, rather than compressing it into one evening meal, as the body can only use a certain amount of protein at any one time and any that isn't used is stored as fat. Try to eat a little at every meal and also aim for two portions of fish each week (one of which should be oily, for the omega 3 benefits). If you're a fan of red meat (I hear you) or processed meat (that phrase makes it sound so unappetising) such as chorizo, try to limit them to around 70 grams a day as they can be high in saturated fats and additives.

EAT FOODS AND DRINKS THAT ARE HIGH IN FAT, SALT AND/OR SUGAR INFREQUENTLY

Most adults and children in the UK are eating too much added sugar. It's nutrient empty, may be addictive, increases our risk of type II diabetes, affects our energy levels and has an overall negative effect on our health. Sugar is often added to processed foods to increase shelf life and to improve taste, and when our diet is so reliant on supermarket convenience foods we are consuming more sugar than we realise. Be aware that many 'low-fat' alternatives (such as low-fat yoghurt) will add sugar to counteract the loss of the flavour and texture the fat would have given. Many of the foods we know to have high sugar (cakes, biscuits, etc.) are often high in fat too. Remember that there are sugars in fruit and milk too, and we call these 'extrinsic sugars' – meaning they are natural to the food. Please don't shy away from fruit because someone's told you it is high in sugar. It's the foods that have sugar added to them that should be kept to a minimum.

When it comes to fat, things are not so simple. There are different types of fat and they all have different effects on the body. There is a whole section on this on page 32 but in summary we should try to limit the levels of saturated fat we consume while unsaturated fats can have many health benefits.

In this book I have included a dessert section. I thought long and hard about my stance on desserts as I felt I should follow the crowd and only choose desserts that were really low in sugar and had lots of other ingredients swapped in to take out the supposed 'bad guys'. When I spoke to the people around me, and my clients, and we shared our experiences of trying 'alternative' desserts, we all had the same stories. We had wanted a slice of cake/brownie/flapjack and instead opted for the 'healthy option' of raw brownies made from air (or similar). We'd eaten more and more of said 'healthy alternative' trying to satisfy the fact that really what we wanted was the cake and, in the end, we may as well have just had the bloody cake. I really feel that a little of what you fancy does you good, so some of the recipes are healthier options and some are simply delicious regular desserts for those times when only cake will do.

One thing we should be mindful of when discussing sugar consumption is emotional eating. It's very rare that when we are sad, or have had a bad day at work, we come home and say, 'Stuart, get me a carrot – I've had a shit day at work'. It tends to be that we get comfort from high-sugar or high-fat foods, due to their links to happy hormones such as dopamine. And while I think it's important to have an outlet to make you feel a little better or happier, it's important to watch out for too much eating for comfort. If you were brought up to see sweets as a reward, it can be a hard habit to break. Just make sure that these foods are eaten infrequently and that they do not become a normal, larger part of your diet.

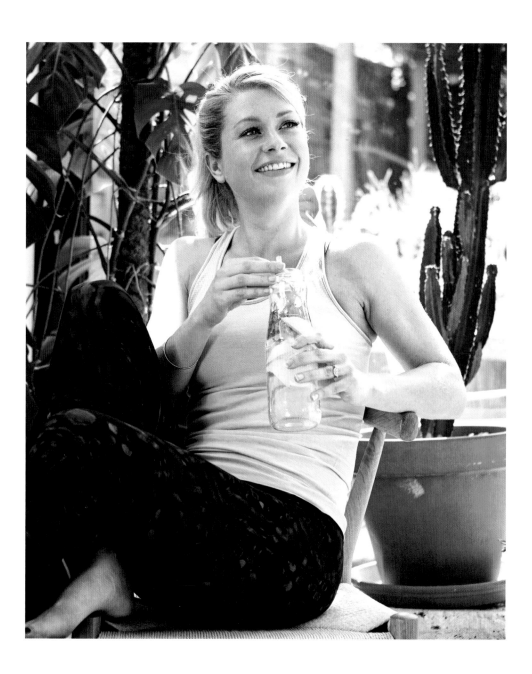

When it comes to reducing sugar, obvious changes are getting rid of sweets, fizzy drinks and 'junk food' from your diet. Replace unhealthy snacks with portions of fruit (remember skin-on is even better). Swap fizzy drinks or fruit juice (which I'm afraid is high in free sugars) with water – you can flavour it yourself with lemon and ginger slices and sprigs of mint, or lime and basil – and choose dark chocolate with a high cocoa content where possible.

DRINK 6–8 CUPS (ABOUT 1.2 LITRES) OF FLUID PER DAY

I mean, this one seems pretty simple. Just drink more water. But it can be easy, during a busy day, to forget. It's really about making it a habit. I feel lost if I don't have a bottle of water on me! Dehydration occurs when your body uses up more liquid than you consume. Remember that we urinate, sweat, poo, lubricate our eyes and mouth, and cry all with our body's water. With water making up over two-thirds of your body, a reduction upsets the balance of minerals and affects how it functions. Water is needed for lubrication of joints and removal of waste products from the body, and it keeps the skin healthy. Digestion relies on water to help bulk out our poos and dehydration can lead to constipation. Dehydration also affects our concentration and energy levels.

All fluids contribute towards your guidelines (except alcohol, I'm afraid) but try not to rely on getting your liquids from caffeine. Six cups of coffee isn't really the solution (plus it'll dehydrate you as it's a diuretic) and fruit juices and soda will add unnecessary sugar to your diet. As I mentioned in the previous section, you can flavour your water really easily if that helps (try not to rely on sugary cordials). Herbs in a bottle of water are delicious and I always start the day with a mug of hot water and lemon juice. If you feel thirsty you are already dehydrated, so try to ensure you are spreading your water consumption out throughout the day – don't leave it until you're already thirsty.

Remember that you must replace the liquids your body uses to avoid dehydration. When we exercise, our body produces sweat to try to cool us down. That sweat is not reabsorbed into the body so you will need to drink more water if you are exercising or it is a hot day. It's wise to ensure you are adequately hydrated before beginning exercise and to take small sips during exercise to keep the body functioning effectively (too much and it'll all come back up again). Some sports drinks can be helpful at replacing electrolytes lost during exercise but many can be full of sugar so be careful or dilute them with extra water if needed.

So there you have it. The main food groups and what the advice is on each. If you've spent the past few years following the newest diets, you've probably spent the past few years being miserable, tired and hungry too. We are so hopeful that someone will come up with a superfood/diet/product/pill that will bypass the need for us to simply eat thoughtfully, but I'm afraid I simply don't believe that will ever happen. We already have all the wonder pills we could ever need and they come in the form of vegetables! Once we realise that there is no shortcut or quick fix, we can start to move on with our lives and make small, obtainable changes. It is important to know what the possible complications associated with a poor diet and lack of exercise are, but again please do not obsess over the number you see on the scales in front of you. It does not define you as a person.

OBESITY – THE FACTS

Obesity is the word on everyone's lips. We can't read a newspaper without seeing the newest headlines about how obese the world is and how much it is costing the NHS in the UK. We're all sat there wondering whether we, or someone we know, are obese and resign ourselves to the fact that the stats show obesity is on the rise. But are we 100 per cent sure what obesity is, or even what the implications really mean? It's the elephant in the room. The million-dollar question: is obesity really that bad?

One in four women in England are currently obese. [13] The figures for obesity rose quite rapidly between 1993 and 2002 but have remained relatively stable since then. However, the prevalence of severe obesity (BMI of 40 and above) has continued to rise.

Let's start with discussing what obesity actually is. Obesity is usually defined using our body mass index (BMI). Our BMI is a number that is calculated using our height and weight. It shows us what weight category we belong to and is widely used by the medical profession. Its strengths are that it is incredibly easy to calculate and relies on no expensive equipment; however, it's accuracy can, albeit rarely, be debatable. First let me show you how you would work out your BMI using the equation below:

Weight in Kilograms ÷ Height in Metres Squared

Another way of expressing this is:

Weight in Kilograms ÷ Height in Metres ÷ Height in Metres

So, if you were to weigh 62 kilograms and were 1.72 metres tall, your BMI would be the following:

62 ÷ 1.72 ÷ 1.72 = 20.9

So we would say that your BMI is 20.9. A BMI below 18.5 is classed as underweight, 18.5–24.9 is considered a 'normal weight', 25.0–29.9 is 'overweight' and 30.0 and above is considered 'obese'.

Now it's really handy having such a simple calculation and lovely clear groups to put us into, but we must remember that humans are not simple creatures and measuring our health is not always as clear cut as putting us through a calculator. The distribution of muscle to fat in our body can very occasionally skew our scores – for example, very large bodybuilders will be heavy and may have a high BMI but that weight will come from muscle, not fat. So can we really say they are obese? Let's be honest, though, how many of us can claim to be a bodybuilder?!

BMI is useful as a general indicator, but it has its limitations. BMI does not tell us about our body's composition. It does not tell us how much body fat we have or what our fitness levels are. It is one metric of health and should really be used in conjunction with others such as blood pressure, cholesterol levels, activity levels and diet. BMI does not tell us what is going on at a cellular level. OK, so we may weigh more than what is considered 'normal', but we may well be healthier than others. You may exercise more, drink less and eat more vegetables, in which case weight does not necessarily determine how healthy you are or how at risk you are of chronic illnesses. In fact, studies have shown that, while being underweight (having a BMI of less than 18.5) or high obesity levels (a BMI higher than 35) does lead to an increase in mortality (rate of death), mortality is actually lower in those who are in the overweight category than in those who are in the normal category. Those in the normal and lower obese (30–35) categories are actually comparable. [14]

So, while we can use BMI as an indication of where we might be in terms of our weight, do not panic and worry that having a BMI that is not considered normal means you are all of a sudden at a huge risk. It is what you put in and what you do with your body that really counts.

One thing you should note: despite studies showing that obesity does not necessarily correlate to mortality, there are links between obesity and morbidity (rate of illness). Specifically, there are links between obesity and heart disease, hypertension and type II diabetes. [15] However, it is hard to say for sure that obesity is the cause of these illnesses as opposed to obesity being a symptom of poor diet or low exercise levels, which in turn may be the actual causes of these illnesses. We must try to improve all health behaviours (cut down on alcohol, quit smoking, participate in exercise and eat to nourish our bodies) to ensure we are doing the best we can to ward off chronic illnesses – not just jumping on the next diet train.

WHAT IS FAT, THEN?

'She's so fat.' 'Do I look fat in this?' 'That'll make you get fat.' 'Is it low fat?' 'I've got a fat ass.' 'We need to fatten you up.' 'I feel so fat at the moment.' 'It's full of fat!' 'What a fat lot of good that was.'

We use the word 'fat' in such a variety of formats that the word has almost lost its meaning. It's such an ugly, abusive word when in fact fat is an important source of energy for us. It's simply the types of fat, and the amounts we are consuming, that can cause health implications. We need to get rid of the negative connotations that are associated with the word and realise that fat is simply a source of energy that, when not used, is stored in our body for later use.

When we eat fat, our body is receiving a rich source of fuel. For every 1 gram of fat consumed, we gain 9 calories worth of energy. That energy fuels your body, and your brain, for its multitude of daily activities plus any extra exercise or exertion you may enjoy. Fat also has a vast range of roles on a cellular level. It builds cell membranes (the 'skin' of each cell) and assists in nerve function (nerves pass information around our bodies). It is required for transporting fat-soluble vitamins (such as A, D and E) around the body to be used elsewhere. It provides us with essential fatty acids, which cannot be made by the body itself and are needed for growth and cell function. All the cells of our body require essential fats to work! It provides warmth to the body and cushions our vital organs to protect them during knocks and falls. That's a lot of positives to come from something we speak so negatively about.

Types of fat can be further broken down into saturated and unsaturated fats. The ratio of each varies from food to food. Products that come from animals, such as meat and dairy products, tend to have higher levels of saturated fats, while fish and nuts are higher in unsaturated fats. The types of fats in what we eat are of great importance as they have very different effects on the body. It is thought that eating a high level of saturated fats has a negative effect on our health as it leads to an increase in cholesterol.

Cholesterol is a lipid (a molecule that is insoluble in water) that is created by the liver, consumed in the food we eat and carried in the blood as a lipoprotein (a lipid attached to a protein). There are two main types of lipoprotein to focus on here. Low-density lipoproteins (LDLs) carry cholesterol around the body to the cells, offering it up to those that might need it. If the cells do not require it, they start to wait around and collect in blood arteries. This collection of cholesterol is harmful to our health. Let's call this type of lipoprotein, very basically, 'bad cholesterol'.

High-density lipoproteins (HDLs), however, are handy things (let's therefore call them 'good cholesterol'). They go around the body looking for cholesterol that's not needed, much like a parent collecting up all of their child's disregarded toys, and take them back to the liver to be broken down and passed out of the body. Higher levels of HDLs are therefore seen as beneficial to the body.

It's thought that eating high levels of saturated fats, smoking and not doing enough exercise all contribute to higher levels of bad cholesterol. Unfortunately, government statistics show that most of us are eating too much saturated fat! Helpfully, it is thought that unsaturated fats contribute to increasing good cholesterol levels, which in turn helps to sweep bad cholesterol out of our bodies.

Unsaturated fats are further broken down into polyunsaturated and monounsaturated fats. Monounsaturated fats are found in certain nuts, such as cashews and peanuts; some oils, such as olive and sesame; and avocados and olives (amongst other sources). Polyunsaturated fats are found in certain seeds, such as pumpkin and sunflower, and nuts, such as pine nuts (my favourite) and walnuts. Two important polyunsaturated fats are omega 3 and omega 6. Most diets are low in omega 3 fats, which are associated with heart health and are found in oily fish, such as mackerel, kippers, salmon and trout. We should be aiming for one to two portions per week of these sources. If you do not eat fish, then flaxseeds and flaxseed oil are a good alternative for omega 3, as are chia seeds, soy beans, walnuts, hemps seeds and tahini (often used in houmous).

All fats are energy dense, meaning we have to do a fair amount of work to use them up. Any fat energy that is not used is stored in the body within the liver and mainly as adipose tissue to be used at a later date. This is your body's way of protecting you and trying to be helpful: imagine if there were all of a sudden a famine – you'd be grateful for those spare fat cells then! Protein and carbohydrates contain less energy (about 4 calories per gram in contrast to the 9 calories per gram in fat), but again any energy not used from these will be stored as fat for later. This is the irony in that we often talk of fat making us fat but in fact too much of any good thing can be bad. If we are overeating frequently, we will store fat no matter what we are eating. The problem is the effect that different types of fat have on your health.

In summary, aim to swap saturated fats (from dairy and meat products) for unsaturated fats (from nuts, seeds and olives) but remember that only 35 per cent of your daily calorie intake should come from fats, so don't overdo it.

VISCERAL FAT AND SUBCUTANEOUS FAT

Energy that is not used up through metabolic processes is stored for later use. When we eat, our body draws as much goodness as it can from the food and takes these nutrients around the body to where they can be used. Fat is broken down into fatty acids, which can make their way in and out of cells to see whether they're needed. Any fatty acids that are not needed bind together to form triglycerides and are stored in fat cells called adipocytes.

When we say that we can 'pinch an inch' or feel 'love handles', what we are really feeling is subcutaneous fat. This is fat that sits under our skin and cushions us and keeps us warm. There is, however, another type of fat that is not so easy to see or feel. Visceral fat is excess intra-abdominal adipose tissue (fat that is stored deep in the abdominal cavity) that sits embedded in the core surrounding our vital organs. Due to its hidden nature, it is not always possible to see if a person has high levels of visceral fat, but it is more common in those who have poor diets and low exercise levels. It is also possible to presume that those with a bigger waistline may have higher levels of visceral fat. This type of fat is seen as far more worrying than subcutaneous fat as it plays a part in altering hormone levels and has been linked to an increased risk of type II diabetes, certain cancers and heart disease. This is another example of the fact that we can't always judge someone's health by how they look or what they weigh. Someone who is slim on the outside can still have high levels of visceral fat.

HELPFUL TIPS TO REDUCE HIGH LEVELS OF VISCERAL FAT

- **Ensure you eat a balanced, nutritious diet.** The key here is 'balanced'. It's about eating the right variety of foods from each food group and nourishing your body.

- **Avoid highly processed and refined foods, especially those high in refined carbohydrates, which cause blood-sugar levels to spike (e.g. sweets, white bread, sugary drinks).** Our bodies are clever and when we are tired or run down they try to encourage us to get our energy from foods that are quick to digest. Foods high in sugar, such as soda, will give us a very quick burst of energy, making us feel incredible, but that energy will not last long. They take next to no time to digest and are absorbed into the blood rapidly. Avoid the trap of getting your energy hits from sugary foods.

- **Make sure you move enough every day.** Lack of exercise causes the body's metabolism to slow down and, if we are not adequately burning the fuel we are consuming, it will be stored for later. Please note that this does not mean you have to go to expensive gyms or run 10 kilometres every day. It can be as simple as going out for a 30 minute walk or doing some housework. Do what you enjoy and you're more likely to stick with it. HIIT has been shown to be effective at reducing body fat and there are various extra benefits to your health that will be discussed in the Sweat chapter, but if you decide you hate it try something else. And keep trying until you find what you love.

- **Try to reduce your stress levels.** High levels of stress cause the hormone cortisol to increase, and cortisol has been linked to an increase in fat stored in the abdomen (visceral fat). Mindfulness is used by many people to help reduce feelings of stress and anxiety, and again exercise is also a great way of shaking off the day's stresses. Ensure you have a good support network around you and try to create a life that is as stress free as possible.

- **Make sure you are sleeping enough – links have been found between lack of sleep and abdominal fat.** Stress, poor diet and lack of exercise can all contribute to poor sleeping patterns so you may find that with a better diet and by moving more your sleep improves. I struggled with simply getting to sleep for a long time when I first started my business as all my creative thoughts and worries seemed to rear their heads at bed time. I have truly benefited from a night-time routine, much like a newborn baby would. If I am particularly stressed, I will practise mindfulness (this is discussed more on page 37). I have a bath, put my pyjamas on, spray my pillow with lavender spray, light a candle, write down any worries or thoughts in my head or in a notepad by my bed, I read for a while (never TV or mindless Instagram trawling) and wear earplugs and an eye mask to sleep. Sleep needs to be seen as vitally important for our health, and I am not willing to compromise. Leave the TV and your phone outside the bedroom. Your bedroom is for two things only and one of them is sleeping.

You might be starting to see a pattern emerge in all the advice that I'm giving you. It always comes back to the same guidelines: move more, eat well and be happy!

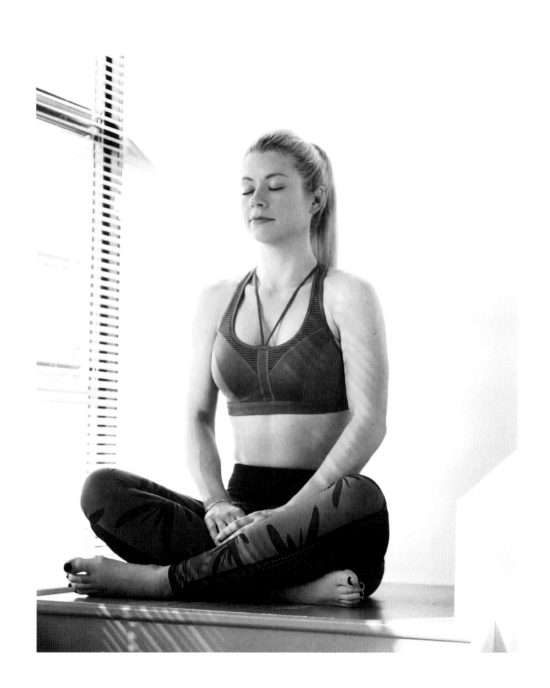

MINDFULNESS: HOW A HEALTHY MIND CREATES A HEALTHY BODY

Ever feel like your day has just rushed by? Like you haven't even had the chance to catch your breath? At my studio, I sometimes sit on the toilet for a few minutes extra just so I can have a rest and a moment's peace. For me, mindfulness has played a huge role in boosting my mood and keeping depression at bay. I have in the past struggled with anxiety and depression and I am always grateful for the skills mindfulness has taught me. You really can't put a price on your health, be it physical or mental, and you don't realise what you have until it's gone. Overwhelming feelings of worry, anxiety and stress can play havoc with an otherwise healthy lifestyle, and eating well and exercising can be the last thing on your mind. If this sounds like you, please give mindfulness a go. It comes into play with the way you eat and the way you move your body throughout this book.

Mindfulness can be described as the state of awareness a person experiences when they bring their attention to the present. It's about bringing your thoughts to the here and now – how your body feels, what your thoughts and feelings are and where you are in space. It can sound a bit odd if it's out of your comfort zone, but essentially it's taking time out of your day to be still and quiet and mindful of what is going on in your mind and body. It doesn't have to be fancy – you don't need to buy a miniature Buddha statue or light incense sticks (although they are freaking relaxing). You can do it anywhere and at any time. It can be practised alone or in a group, seated or lying, and in silence or through guided meditation (someone talking you through your practice).

Mindfulness has been around for many years and is thought to originate in the teachings of the Buddha. It has been adapted over the years, with more and more research taking place into the effects it has on our health and happiness. The research has increasingly found that those who regularly practise mindfulness techniques experience less stress, anxiety and depression. [16] It is increasingly recommended for those who have suffered depression to prevent relapse, and more and more people are opening their minds to the benefits it may bring.

Mindfulness can take various forms, not simply the acts described above. Mindfulness when walking, exercising and eating all come back to the process of paying attention to how our bodies feel, what our minds think and what emotions we experience during the task.

MINDFUL EATING

Whenever I go to get waxed (too much information?) I lie there looking through Instagram. Why? Not because I have some creepy tendencies, but because it takes my mind off the pain I am experiencing. Looking at the beautiful images and reading the hilarious comments makes the whole process forgettable and seem much quicker. It's the same as when the dentist puts a TV on the ceiling for you to watch antiques programmes while you're having a root canal – it seems to make it that bit less painful.

So imagine what happens when you eat your dinner in front of the TV. Hopefully by the end of this book, you will be spending enjoyable time sourcing, smelling and tasting your ingredients. You will put love into your meal and relish the end product. You will serve it up beautifully and, if you're eating with someone else, you'll present it to them with pride.

For many of us, you'll sit and mindlessly eat your meal while concentrating fully on the TV. By the end of it, you won't even be able to remember what you've just eaten, let alone what it tasted like. It's over in an instant and you feel completely unsatisfied. When you eat mindlessly rather than mindfully, it is a waste of all your effort and a challenge for your digestive system.

When we eat, a complex combination of hormones stimulate the gut to prepare it for digesting food. The gut is prepared for food that has begun the breakdown process in the mouth and is suitably chewed. It can take a while for our body to recognise it is full and does not require extra food – often longer than it has taken you to finish your meal. The problem with eating while not paying full attention to what we are doing is we end up chewing less and eating faster than we should. If we eat too quickly, our body does not yet realise it has had enough food, and overeating will ensue as we reach for seconds. The gut struggles to break down food that has not been properly chewed and, if it is rushed down too quickly, indigestion can cause discomfort as the body struggles to process your meal. Poor digestion prevents us from fully extracting the correct nutrients from our food – so all your efforts to nourish your body could go to waste.

There is also the possibility that carrying out other activities may divert the blood flow away from the gut to elsewhere at a time when it is needed for digestion. If we are concentrating on something else, especially if it is energetic or stressful, our body is in its 'fight or flight' mode. In this mode the body is trying to conserve its energy, and digesting food is not on its agenda at all.

All in all, eating while distracted is not enjoyable or healthy for the body and we are more likely to overeat or make poor food choices.

TIPS TO MINDFULLY ENJOY YOUR FOOD

- **Focus on the task ahead.** You have one task right now and that is to eat, and enjoy, your food. Switch off the TV, put your phone on silent and get rid of the radio – simply sit and concentrate on what you are doing. Focus your mind on how your food tastes, what the textures are and what you can smell.

- **Chew your food.** Take smaller bites and really chew your food. The more you do in the mouth, the less taxing it will be on your gut. The enzymes in your mouth help to start the process of breaking down your food, so take the pressure off your gut and chew, chew, chew.

- **Check in with your body.** Are you actually hungry? Or are you bored? Or emotional? Start to tune in to your body's natural hunger. We are often led to eat by the time of day or the limitations we have at work. This means a lot of us have forgotten what hunger really feels like. If you're unsure why you are opening the fridge, go read a book or go for a walk and see whether you are still hungry.

- **Think about where your food has come from.** Try to imagine the journey your food has taken. Where did it start? Where was it grown? How was it cooked? This will give you a greater appreciation of what your food means to you and how lucky you are to get to enjoy it. Remember we want to have positive feelings towards food!

- **Be realistic.** As much as it would be lovely to have an hour of silence to eat our meals in, this just isn't always realistic. Some of you will have children who want to tell you how their day was, and some of you might work long hours and need to multitask. I am not saying you have to do this all the time – I am definitely guilty of eating a tin of tuna in 20 seconds between clients – but even if the odd meal is eaten without distraction then that can only be a good thing. You could even stop half-way through a meal and quickly check in with whether you are still enjoying it or still hungry. Don't stress about it and don't force it, but give it a go when you can.

EATING SEASONALLY

Eating with the seasons is not only cost effective but also far better for the environment (and us). At present, the UK imports a large proportion of its fruit and vegetables from abroad. This is simply down to the fact that we want the convenience of having access to all foods at all times. But the cost to the environment is undeniable, as produce is flown, shipped and driven to its new home. Moreover, it can take a long time for the produce to make it to you and as time goes on the nutrients can deplete.

If you want to eat raspberries in January, you'll have no chance finding fresh ones in the UK – it's too cold – so you'll have no option but to buy ones that have been imported from Spain. Buying frozen produce is a great way to eat out of season. But, instead of the raspberries, why not have some rhubarb? If we can be a little more inventive, and mindful of what is in season, we may be able to spend less, help the environment and support our local community. Please do not think this is me saying you are bad if you eat imported fruit and vegetables – it is almost impossible not to do so, and if eating that Indian mango means you're trying more fruit then that is a good thing! I'm just talking about being a little bit more aware of where your food comes from.

Although not exhaustive, the page opposite lists the seasonal produce available each month. I hope it inspires you!

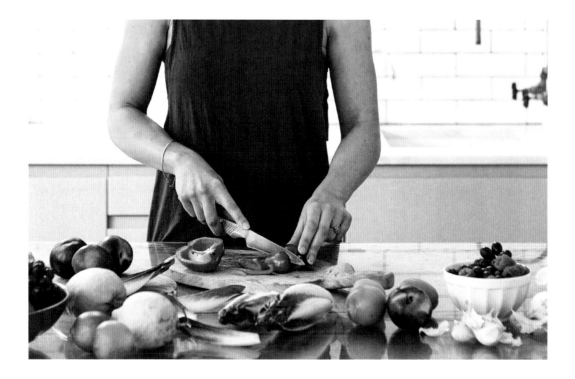

Month	Seasonal produce list
JANUARY	Apples, beetroots, brussels sprouts, cabbages, carrots, chicory, Jerusalem artichokes, kale, parsnips, pears, squash, swedes, turnips
FEBRUARY	Apples, beetroots, brussels sprouts, cabbages, carrots, chicory, Jerusalem artichokes, kale, onions, parsnips, pears, purple sprouting broccoli, squash, swedes
MARCH	Artichokes, beetroots, cabbages, carrots, chicory, cucumbers, parsnips, purple sprouting broccoli, radishes, rhubarb, watercress
APRIL	Artichokes, beetroots, cabbages, carrots, chicory, kale, new potatoes, parsnips, radishes, rhubarb, rocket, spinach, watercress
MAY	Artichokes, asparagus, aubergines, beetroots, chicory, elderflowers, lettuce, new potatoes, peas, peppers, radishes, rhubarb, rocket, spinach, strawberries, watercress
JUNE	Asparagus, aubergines, beetroots, blackcurrants, broad beans, broccoli, cauliflowers, cherries, chicory, courgettes, cucumber, elderflowers, gooseberries, lettuce, new potatoes, peas, peppers, radishes, raspberries, rhubarb, rocket, runner beans, strawberries, summer squash, Swiss chard, turnips, watercress
JULY	Aubergine, beetroots, blackberries, blackcurrants, blueberries, broad beans, broccoli, carrots, cauliflowers, cherries, chicory, courgettes, cucumbers, gooseberries, fennel, French beans, new potatoes, onions, peas, potatoes, radishes, raspberries, redcurrants, rhubarb, rocket, runner beans, strawberries, summer squash, Swiss chard, tomatoes, turnips, watercress
AUGUST	Aubergine, beetroots, blackberries, blackcurrants, broad beans, broccoli, carrots, cauliflowers, cherries, courgettes, cucumbers, fennel, French beans, leeks, lettuce, mangetout, parsnips, peas, peppers, potatoes, plums, pumpkins, radishes, raspberries, redcurrants, rhubarb, rocket, runner beans, strawberries, summer squash, sweetcorn, Swiss chard, tomatoes, watercress
SEPTEMBER	Aubergines, beetroots, blackberries, broccoli, brussels sprouts, butternut squash, carrots, cauliflowers, courgettes, cucumbers, kale, leeks, lettuce, mangetout, parsnips, pears, peas, peppers, plums, potatoes, pumpkins, radishes, raspberries, rhubarb, rocket, runner beans, spinach, strawberries, summer squash, sweetcorn, Swiss chard, tomatoes, turnips, watercress
OCTOBER	Aubergines, apples, beetroots, blackberries, broccoli, brussels sprouts, butternut squash, carrots, cauliflowers, chestnuts, courgettes, cucumbers, kale, parsnips, pears, peas, potatoes, pumpkins, radishes, rocket, runner beans, spinach, summer squash, swede, sweetcorn, Swiss chard, tomatoes, turnips, watercress, winter squash
NOVEMBER	Apples, beetroots, brussels sprouts, butternut squash, cabbages, carrots, cauliflowers, chestnuts, cranberries, elderberries, Jerusalem artichokes, kale, leeks, parsnips, pears, potatoes, pumpkins, swede, Swiss chard, turnips, watercress, winter squash
DECEMBER	Apples, beetroots, brussels sprouts, carrots, chestnuts, chicory, cranberries, Jerusalem artichokes, kale, parsnips, pears, potatoes, pumpkins, red cabbages, swede, Swiss chard, turnips, watercress, winter squash

YOUR NOURISH RECIPES

So now for the bit you've all been waiting for, and hopefully haven't just skipped straight to (if you have, go back – there's really important information in this chapter!). The recipes. These recipes have not been created to be specifically low fat, or low carb, or low calorie. We've all tried that and it's not worked. These are more about adding *in* to our diets. About getting more vegetables, more fibre, more nutrients into our bodies and getting more enjoyment out of cooking. If you even swap one ready meal for one of my recipes or try a new vegetable from this book, I'll be happy.

All of these recipes have been assessed by nutritionist Laura Thomas, PhD., and have been enjoyed by myself, my husband and our friends. I have chosen not to list their calorie content for the same reasons I give in this chapter. Obsessing over calorie counting has done us no favours over the years and can lead to disordered eating. Instead try to eat a varied diet – don't just eat the Squash and Rosemary Carbonara (see page 83) every night (although it's pretty tempting, and when creating these recipes I ate it three times in one week) – and try to check in with how each recipe makes you feel. Do you feel energised after or tired? Has it helped you feel 'more regular' or do you feel bloated? It's your body – take ownership of what you choose to put in it.

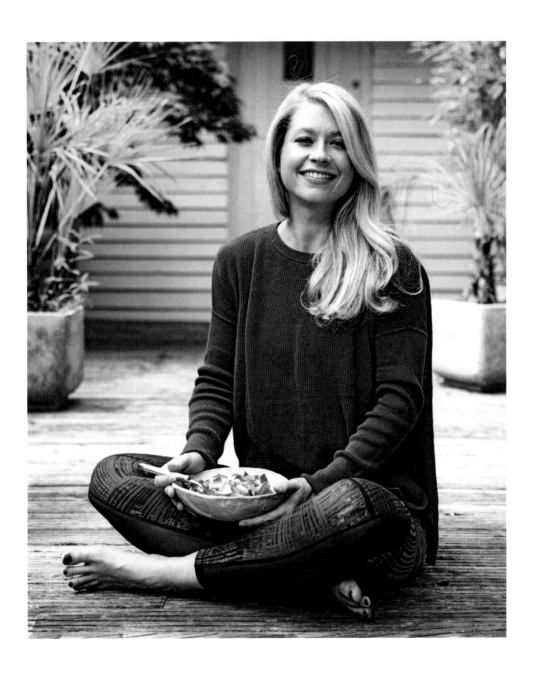

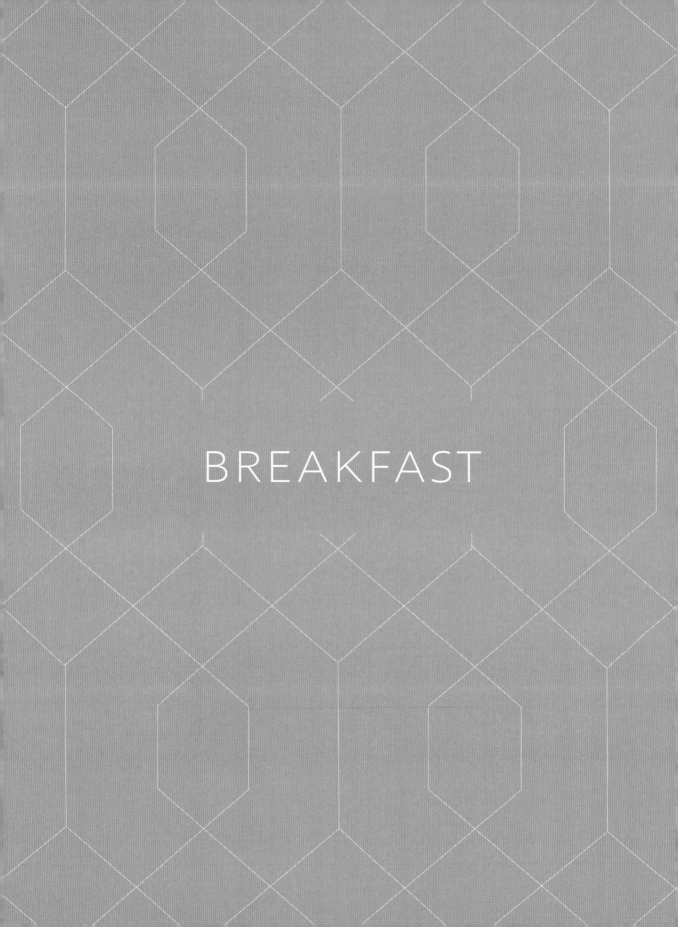

BREAKFAST

BANANA AND OAT ENERGY BARS

MAKES 8 BARS

These bars are great to wrap up and take to work if you are in a rush.
I also eat them as a mid-morning snack or after a workout to give me
a boost. Oats are a great source of fibre, and bananas are a source of
potassium, which our muscles need to function properly.

1 tbsp coconut oil
or butter, plus extra
for greasing

1½ tbsp honey

4 ripe bananas,
peeled and mashed

11 dried apricots,
roughly chopped

10 prunes, roughly
chopped

60g sultanas

10g dried
cranberries

160g porridge oats

Preheat the oven to 160°C Fan (180°C/350°F/Gas Mark 4) and grease a
brownie tin with oil. Any square or rectangular tin with high sides will do.

Melt the oil or butter and honey together in a large saucepan then remove
from the heat. Stir in the rest of the ingredients and mix well.

Spoon the mixture into the greased brownie tin. It doesn't need to fill the
tin completely, just push it into a square shape about 3cm thick – it won't
spread in the oven.

Bake in the oven for 20–25 minutes, until the top of the mixture has
slightly darkened.

Remove the tin from the oven and cut the mixture into bars in the tin
while the mixture is still warm, then leave to cool.

The bars will keep for up to a week in a sealed container in the fridge.

Tips:
If you are gluten intolerant, use gluten-free oats.
If you are vegan, swap the honey for maple syrup.

BAKED BLACK BEANS, CORIANDER GUACAMOLE AND POACHED EGGS

SERVES 4

I first had a dish like this in a café in Bristol. The beans were spicy, the guacamole was fragrant and it was topped with a perfect poached egg. Black beans are high in both protein and fibre, and fibre plays an important role in digestive health and can help with bowel function.

White wine vinegar

4 eggs

For the black beans:

Small knob of butter or 1 tsp olive oil

1 carrot, peeled and finely chopped

1 onion, finely chopped

1 celery stick, finely chopped

$^1/_3$ fresh red chilli, finely chopped

1 garlic clove, finely chopped

200ml chicken (or vegetable) stock

1 bay leaf

400g tin of black beans, drained and rinsed

400g tin of good-quality chopped tomatoes

½ tsp ground cumin

½ tsp hot paprika

Sea salt and freshly ground black pepper

To make the baked black beans, melt the butter (or heat the oil) in a large saucepan over a medium heat, add the carrot, onion, celery and chilli and fry for 5 minutes, until the onions are soft. Add the rest of the ingredients, season with salt and pepper, bring to the boil, then simmer gently for 15 minutes (or longer, if you have the time – the longer you simmer the beans, the better their flavour), adding water if the sauce starts to dry out.

Meanwhile, make the guacamole. Mash the avocado in a large bowl, add the remaining ingredients, season with salt and pepper and cover the bowl with cling film until needed.

Just before the beans are ready, poach the eggs. Bring a pan of water to the boil over a high heat and add a splash of vinegar. Reduce the heat to a simmer. Crack one egg at a time into a coffee mug, then carefully tip each egg into the water (turning up the heat if the water stops simmering). Leave the eggs to simmer for 2–3 minutes.

Ladle the beans into bowls, add a dollop of guacamole to each serving and top with a drained poached egg, a sprinkle of chilli flakes and fresh coriander.

For the guacamole:

2 ripe avocados, peeled and stoned

3 spring onions, thinly sliced

Pinch of dried chilli flakes, plus extra to serve

Squeeze of lime juice

Small bunch of fresh coriander, chopped, plus extra to serve

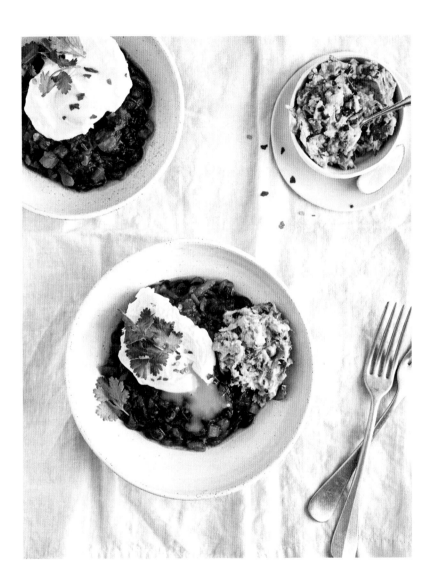

Tips:

Other beans, such as borlotti or red kidney beans, work just as well as black beans in this recipe.

The baked beans can also be made up to a day in advance and reheated when needed.

You can deseed your chilli if you don't like your food too spicy.

VANILLA MULTIGRAIN PORRIDGE

SERVES 1

Porridge is one of the simplest, quickest and most filling breakfasts out there. This version combines the benefits of two grains and one seed to create a nourishing breakfast that is a good source of fibre. The barley and oats contain beta-glucans which help maintain normal blood cholesterol.

Leaving the mixture to soak overnight makes it quicker to cook and will save you time in the morning.

20g buckwheat groats

20g quick-cook barley

20g porridge oats

250ml almond milk (or oat, rice, coconut or cow's milk)

Seeds scraped from a 3cm piece of vanilla pod (pod retained)

1 tsp good-quality honey (optional)

Rinse the buckwheat groats and barley thoroughly in a sieve under cold running water, drain and put them into a small bowl. Add the oats, milk, vanilla seeds, plus the empty pod. Stir, cover and place in the fridge overnight.

In the morning, pour the mixture into a small saucepan, add the honey, if using, and simmer gently for about 5 minutes or until thick. You can always add a splash of water if you want to make it runnier. Remove the vanilla pod, pour the porridge into a bowl, top with your favourite fruit compote and sprinkle with chopped nuts.

Tips:

To make this gluten-free, simply use gluten-free oats, remove the barley and use double the quantity of the oats.

If you are vegan, feel free to swap the honey for an alternative natural sweetener and use your favourite nut milk.

SAVOURY THYME PORRIDGE
with Sautéed Mushrooms and Walnuts

SERVES 1

If you haven't tried savoury porridge yet, bear with me. It may sound odd but it is incredibly tasty and I really like starting the day with something savoury rather than sweet (there is no added sugar in this recipe). I love to top it with a fried egg, cooked in a little butter. Make sure you use jumbo oats and fry the mushrooms until they are dark brown and slightly crisp. Rosemary is equally delicious in this (in place of the thyme).

2 tsp butter or olive oil

2 chestnut mushrooms, thinly sliced

1cm piece of fresh red chilli, chopped

1 thyme sprig, leaves picked

1 small onion, chopped

60g jumbo porridge oats

300ml chicken (or vegetable) stock

1 egg (optional)

2 walnuts, crushed

Freshly ground black pepper

Melt half the butter (or heat the oil) in a large frying pan over a high heat and, once hot, gently lay the sliced mushrooms in the pan, flat-side down. Leave to fry, untouched, for a minute then flip over. If it's golden brown and slightly crisp they are all ready to flip. If not, leave for a further 30 seconds then flip them over. When both sides are deep brown, add the chilli and thyme, give the mushrooms a final stir then reduce the heat to low.

Melt the remaining butter (or heat the oil) in a medium saucepan, add the onion and sauté until soft. Add the oats and stock and bring to a gentle simmer.

Move your mushrooms to one side of the frying pan, increase the heat and crack the egg into the pan, if using. Fry until crispy around the edges.

Once the oats are soft and the stock has been absorbed, pour the porridge into a bowl, top with the mushrooms, walnuts and fried egg, and finish with some freshly ground black pepper.

Tips:

If you are gluten intolerant you can use gluten-free oats and stock.

If you are vegan, use vegetable stock and swap the egg for extra mushrooms.

CORN AND LIME FRITTERS
with Avocado, Rocket and Sriracha Sauce

SERVES 2

Corn fritters are so delicious! The batter takes just a few minutes to mix up and they need only five minutes in the pan. The lime zest cuts through the creaminess of the corn and the sriracha adds some heat. Flaxseed helps to increase the fibre content of the dish, which is also a source of protein. All in all, the recipe contributes to at least two of your five-a-day.

Large handful of rocket

1 ripe avocado, peeled, stoned and flesh sliced

Sriracha sauce (optional)

Juice of ½ lime

Small handful of fresh coriander

Sea salt and freshly ground black pepper

For the fritters:

165g tin of sweetcorn, drained

5 spring onions, thinly sliced

1 egg

1 tbsp plain flour

1 heaped tsp ground flaxseed

½ tsp hot smoked paprika

Small handful of fresh coriander, chopped

Grated zest of ½ lime

1 tbsp olive oil

Mix all the ingredients for the fritters together (except the oil) in a bowl with a pinch of salt and pepper and stir well. Leave for up to 5 minutes so the mixture binds better when cooked.

Heat the oil in a large frying pan over a high heat. When hot, pour half the batter mixture into the pan to create a round fritter, flattening it slightly as you go to create a disk of around 2.5cm thick. Repeat with the other half of the mixture.

After a few minutes, when the underside of each fritter is golden brown, carefully flip them over and cook on the other side for a few minutes. Once they are golden on both sides, transfer the fritters to a plate lined with kitchen paper to absorb any excess oil.

Place the fritters on separate plates, top with rocket, slices of avocado and a squirt of sriracha, if you like, and serve with the lime juice, fresh coriander and some black pepper.

Tips:

You can find flaxseed in your local health-food store or online. It's a great way of increasing your fibre intake and can be added to most recipes without affecting the flavour.

Feel free to swap the rocket for spinach, and gluten-free flour works perfectly in place of the plain flour, if needed.

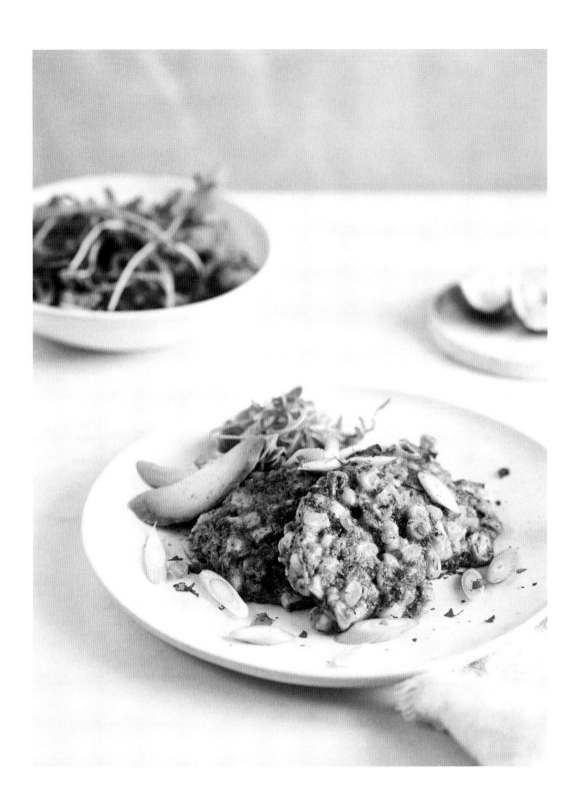

ORANGE AND SEA SALT GRANOLA
with Cashew and Cacao Nibs

SERVES 6–8

This granola is high in fibre, filling and will satisfy those with a sweet tooth. I keep a small pot in my handbag to use as trail mix when I'm on the go. It keeps well in a sealed jar for a week or two (if it's not eaten by then!) and the nuts keep me feeling fuller for longer than other cereals do. I try to bake some each Sunday for the week ahead and it's great for a speedy breakfast.

100g coconut oil

100g honey

Grated zest of ½ orange

Seeds from ½ vanilla pod (optional)

75g sunflower seeds

75g pumpkin seeds

100g cashews

250g porridge oats

1 heaped tsp sea salt

50g cacao nibs

Preheat the oven to 160°C Fan (180°C/350°F/Gas Mark 4) and line two baking sheets with greaseproof paper.

Melt the coconut oil and honey in a small saucepan then remove the pan from the heat and add the orange zest and vanilla seeds, if using.

Mix the seeds, nuts, oats and salt together in a large bowl then pour the honey and coconut oil into the bowl and mix well.

Divide the mixture between the two baking sheets, spread it out evenly and bake in the oven for 10–15 minutes, until golden brown, turning the mixture every 5 minutes.

Remove from the oven and leave the granola to cool on the sheets then add the cacao nibs and tip the granola into a large jar.

Tips:

If you are gluten intolerant, there are great gluten-free oats available in most stores now. Organic oats are not much more expensive than regular oats, so I like to use them in this recipe where possible. Feel free to swap the seeds and nuts for ones you prefer.

If you are vegan, swap the honey for maple syrup. Remember that the chemical structure of all sugars is the same so there is nothing necessarily wrong with using golden syrup if this is all you have.

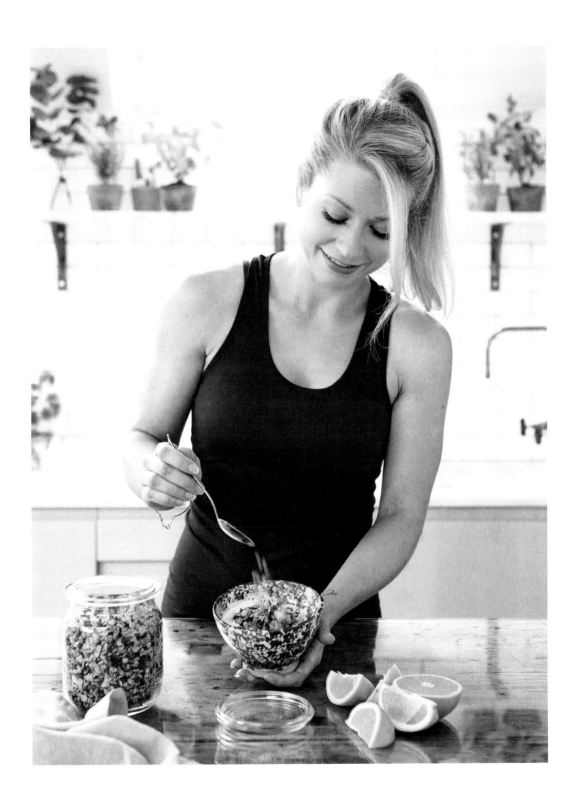

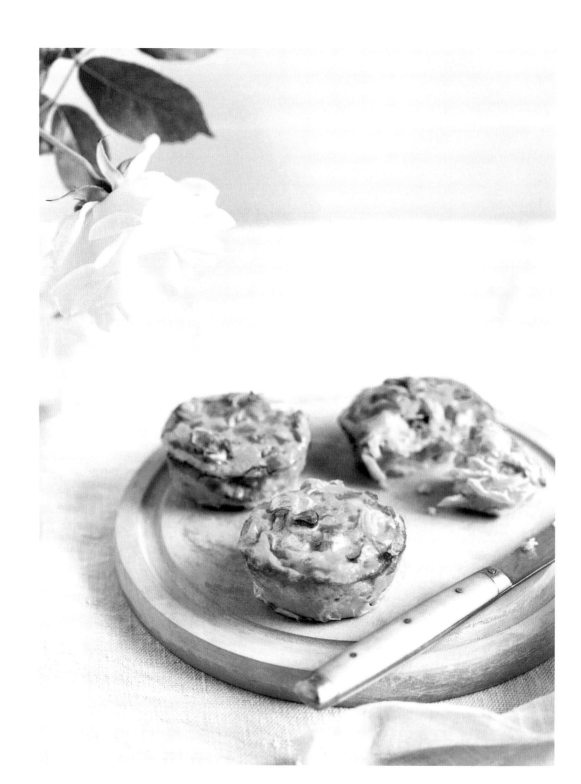

SMOKED SALMON, EGG AND TURMERIC MUFFINS

MAKES 4

These protein-rich, no-added-sugar muffins are easy to make and can be cooked the night before, to take to work the next day. They are equally nice with feta cheese instead of the salmon and you can swap in your favourite veggies, too. Feel free to experiment – sweetcorn and cherry tomatoes with fresh chilli is delicious!

½ tsp olive oil

2 small slices of smoked salmon, each cut in half

3 spring onions, thinly sliced

3 large eggs

Splash of milk

2 tsp turmeric

½ tsp hot smoked paprika

½ red pepper, finely chopped

Pinch of cracked black pepper

Preheat the oven to 160°C Fan (180°C/350°F/Gas Mark 4) and grease four holes in a muffin tin with the oil.

Lay a small piece of smoked salmon around the bottom of each greased muffin hole, pressing them flat.

Whisk together the rest of the ingredients in a small bowl and carefully pour the mixture into the muffin holes. You can fill the holes quite high but be careful as you transfer them to the oven.

Bake for about 13 minutes, or until a skewer inserted into the centre of one of the muffins comes out clean. Try not to open the oven door until they are almost ready as they can collapse if brought out before being cooked through. Remove the tin from the oven, carefully run a knife around the edge of each muffin while they're still hot, and carefully lift them out onto a plate.

Tip:
Herbs such as rosemary and thyme go beautifully with eggs and I love adding a sprinkle of luxurious truffle salt to the mix if we have friends visiting.

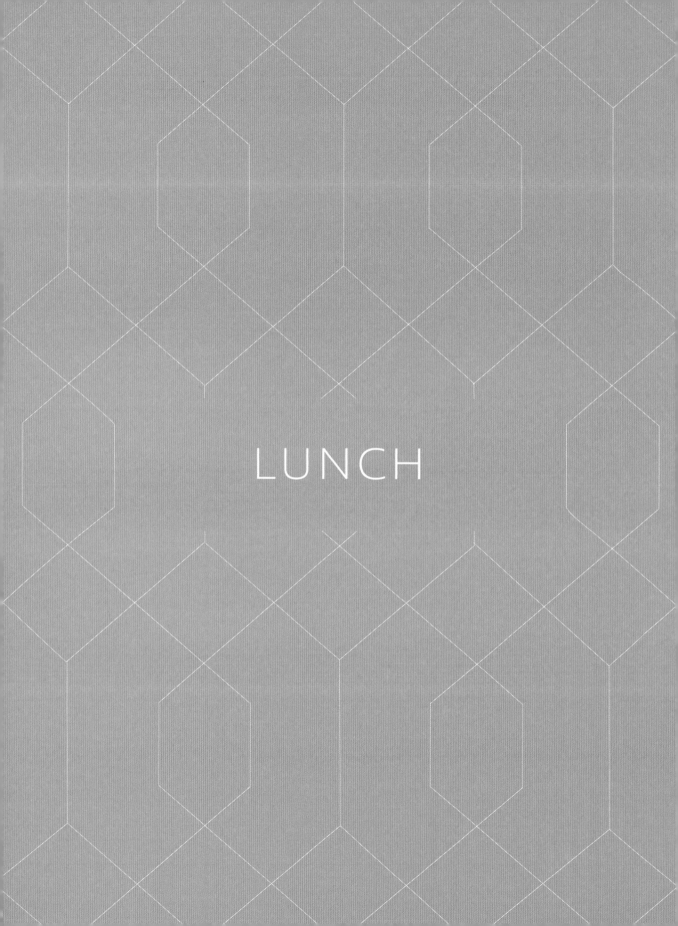

LUNCH

CHORIZO, BUTTERBEAN, SPELT AND KALE BROTH

SERVES 2

This soup takes only 20 minutes to make and can be made the night before and reheated the next day (it's a great one to take to work). If you can't find quick-cook spelt, regular spelt is fine but you will need to cook the soup for around 30 minutes longer. This recipe is a good source of protein and a source of fibre.

Knob of butter or 1 tbsp olive oil

2 leeks, washed and sliced

2 celery sticks, sliced

75g soft cooking chorizo, diced

10 thyme sprigs, leaves picked

Pinch of dried chilli flakes

Pinch of freshly ground black pepper

700ml chicken stock (low-salt if possible)

60g quick-cook spelt

200g tinned butterbeans, drained and rinsed

Melt the butter (or heat the oil) in a large saucepan over a medium heat.

Add the leeks, celery and chorizo and cook for 5 minutes, until the leeks are soft. Add the rest of the ingredients and simmer for 10 minutes. The spelt should be al dente, the soup spicy and the beans warm.

Tips:

Chorizo can be quite salty, as can stock, so avoid adding any further salt to the soup. There are low-sodium stocks available which I much prefer to use over regular stock.

If you are vegan, feel free to swap the chorizo for ½ teaspoon of smoked hot paprika and use vegetable stock instead.

Wholegrain pasta can be swapped in for the spelt if you prefer, or if you are struggling to find spelt in shops.

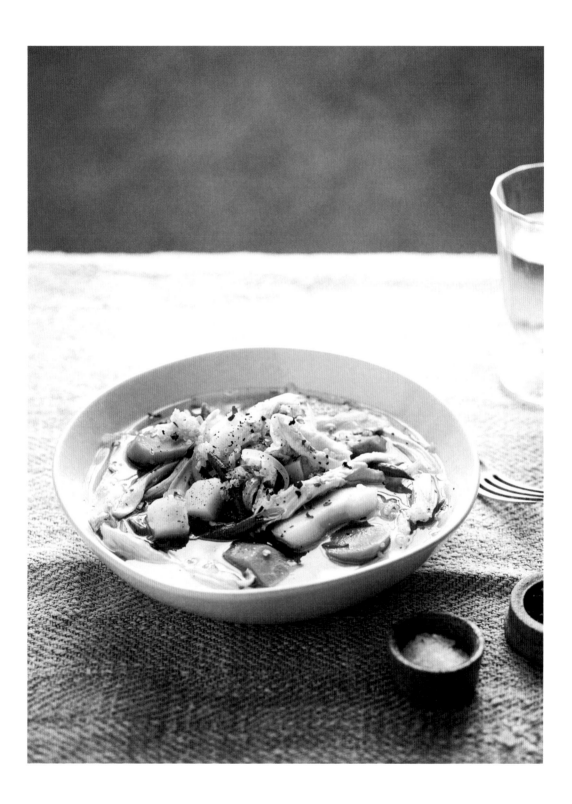

WARMING CHICKEN STEW
with Quinoa, Chilli and Winter Vegetables

SERVES 4

My mum has always made chicken stew with the carcass from our Sunday roast. We would never dream of throwing the bones away and my friends have often thought me mad for boiling a carcass for hours on a Sunday night. The results are delicious though, and this stew is a good source of vitamin A which is great for the skin, eyes and immune system. Throw in any vegetables you have left in your fridge and even make use of leftover cooked vegetables from a roast (they will take less time to cook). You can eat the stew straight away, but I like to take it to work in a box as it tastes even better warmed up the next day.

1 large roast chicken carcass (and whatever is left of your roast chicken)

2 medium white onions, thinly sliced

3 large carrots, peeled and thickly sliced

1 large parsnip, peeled and thickly sliced

1 large potato, peeled and cubed

100g quinoa (or brown rice), rinsed

Pinch of dried chilli flakes

2 large handfuls of green beans, halved widthways

Salt and freshly ground black pepper

To make the broth, place the carcass, leftover meat and any juices (which will resemble jelly) in a large saucepan. Pour in enough cold water to completely cover the chicken (plus a bit more). Bring to the boil, cover, then reduce to a simmer and cook for 3–4 hours, until the carcass has fallen apart and a broth has formed.

Strain the broth into a bowl, jug or pan to remove the bones, then pour the strained broth back into the large saucepan.

Once your carcass has cooled slightly, pick off all the leftover chicken and add it to the pan of broth. You can now throw away the bones.

Add all the other ingredients, except the beans, to the pan, season with salt and pepper and simmer for about 25 minutes, until the carrots are soft and the potatoes and quinoa (or rice) cooked through.

Add the beans and simmer for a further 5 minutes then pour the stew into large bowls, adding a final grind of black pepper.

Tips:

You can add extra cooked chicken if you have very little left on your carcass.

To make this extra special you could add a handful of fried bacon lardons to the mixture.

THAI SLAW SALAD
with Chicken and Cashews

SERVES 2

This really quick salad is a good source of protein and is a great way to use up leftover meat from your roast chicken (see page 71). It can be made the night before and taken to work for lunch, but I keep the sauce mix in a separate jar as it will start to break down the cabbage if left on the slaw overnight. This dish is equally delicious with fresh king prawns or salmon.

¹/₃ white cabbage, thinly sliced with a mandoline (or by hand)

½ red onion, thinly sliced with a mandoline (or by hand)

1 tsp fish sauce

2 tsp sesame oil

Juice of ½ lime

½ fresh red chilli, thinly sliced

2 handfuls of leftover roast chicken (or other shop-bought cooked chicken)

Small handful of sesame seeds

Small handful of cashews or peanuts, slightly crushed

Handful of fresh coriander, chopped

Combine the cabbage and onion in a large bowl to make your salad base.

In a separate small bowl whisk together the fish sauce, sesame oil, lime juice and chilli, then pour it over your salad (if eating straight away) and mix well. If you're making the salad in advance, store the sauce in a jar in the fridge until ready to serve.

Divide the salad between two bowls, top with the chicken, seeds, crushed cashews and coriander, and serve.

Tip:
If you don't like fish sauce (it can be quite pungent) swap it for an equal measure of soy sauce.

FIG, MOZZARELLA AND CANDIED WALNUT SALAD

SERVES 2

I adore figs. They always add impact to a dish and, when soft, have the most incredible sweetness. This dish looks beautiful but in fact takes very little effort or time to make. It can be taken to work easily or used as a side dish for other meals.

10 walnuts

2 tsp honey

4 ripe figs, cut into quarters

1 tsp olive oil

60g watercress

10 basil leaves

½ lemon

1 mozzarella ball, torn into small chunks

Preheat the oven to 180°C Fan (200°C/400°F/Gas Mark 6) and line a roasting tray with foil.

Heat a small saucepan over a medium heat, add the walnuts and half the honey and gently fry the nuts for 2 minutes until they are sticky and caramelised. Transfer them to a bowl and pop them in the fridge until needed.

Lay the figs on the lined roasting tray. Drizzle the oil and remaining honey across the figs and roast in the oven for 8–10 minutes, or until soft.

Divide the watercress and basil leaves between two large plates. Squeeze the juice from the lemon over them and top each plate of leaves with the torn mozzarella. Add the roasted figs and candied walnuts, and serve.

Tip:

You can swap the mozzarella for goats' cheese or feta if you prefer, and swap the basil for mint.

THE NOURISH BOWL

SERVES 2

This is, quite simply, a combination of some of my favourite foods. I crave this when I am ill, hungover, or run down, which I can only presume is a good thing. It can seem a bit of a faff to make all the elements but it doesn't have to take long and you can always double up some of the elements and use them the following day. Simply stack all the ingredients in two bowls and serve. It's a great source of fibre, low in saturated fat and sugar, and a good source of protein.

For the green lentil, garlic and chilli falafels:

400g tin of cooked green lentils, drained, rinsed and left to dry out slightly

1 garlic clove, crushed

½ fresh red chilli

1 heaped tbsp plain flour

1 tbsp olive oil

Salt and freshly cracked black pepper

Put the lentils, garlic and chilli in a blender or food processor, add a small pinch of salt and a large pinch of cracked black pepper and pulse a couple of times. You don't want a paste, so don't over-blend the mixture. Transfer the mixture to a bowl and stir in the flour.

Heat the olive oil in a large frying pan over a medium heat. When hot, scoop up a tablespoonful of mixture, press it together to bind it slightly, then carefully place it in the pan. Repeat with the rest of the mixture – you should have 6–8 patties. Carefully place the patties in the hot oil and fry for about 5 minutes, until golden brown on one side, then turn them and fry them for a further 5 minutes until golden brown all over. Remove from the pan and transfer the patties to a plate lined with kitchen paper to soak up any excess oil.

Serve the falafels with:

2 tbsp Aubergine and Harissa Hummus (page 93)

1 portion of Apricot, Mint and Pistachio Quinoa (page 98)

1 portion of Beetroot, Orange and Poppy Seed Salad (page 99)

2 tbsp Sauerkraut (optional)

4 radishes, sliced

Large handful of rocket

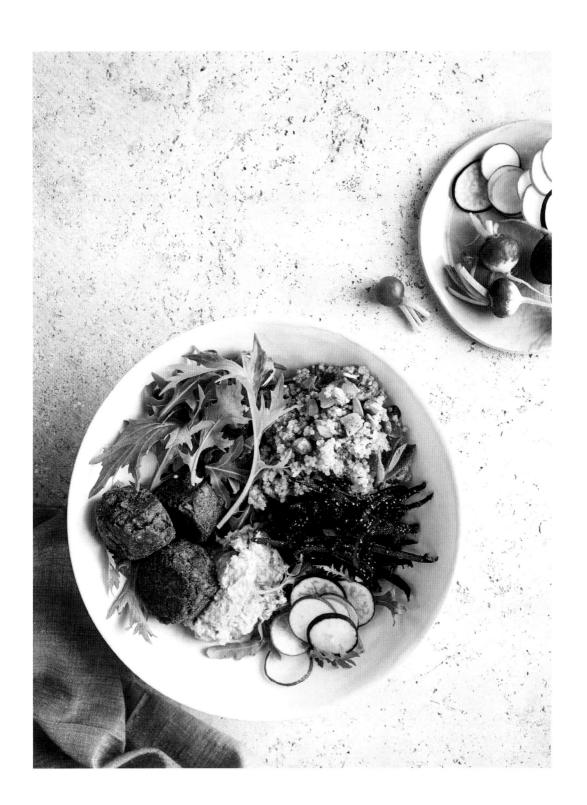

CHICKPEA AND CORIANDER FALAFEL WRAPS

with Sweet Chilli Sauce and Cream Cheese

SERVES 4

I love falafels but sometimes find them a little dry. By mashing the falafel ingredients slightly, rather than blitzing them in a food processor, you can avoid this and keep them moist. The sweet chilli sauce is a welcome addition and chickpeas are a source of protein. This recipe is also a source of fibre (corn tortillas contain more fibre than wheat flour tortillas). You can easily make these at home for lunch or dinner and take any leftovers to work the next day. Try making them for your Nourish bowl too (see page 62), in place of the lentil falafel.

For the falafels:

2 x 400g tins of chickpeas, drained and rinsed

10 spring onions, thinly sliced

1 heaped tsp flaxseed meal (ground flaxseeds)

1 fresh red chilli, deseeded and chopped

Small handful of fresh coriander, chopped

1 egg, plus 1 egg yolk

1 tbsp olive oil

Sea salt and freshly ground black pepper

For the sweet chilli sauce:

3 tbsp honey

½ fresh red chilli, finely chopped

Bring a large saucepan of water to the boil, add the chickpeas and simmer for 10 minutes, then drain and tip them into a large bowl. Add the rest of the falafel ingredients (except the olive oil), season with salt and pepper and, using a potato masher, break the mixture down a little – you don't want it to be smooth or resemble a paste, you just want it to stick together.

Heat the olive oil in a large frying pan over a medium heat. When hot, scoop up a tablespoonful of mixture, press it together to bind it slightly, then carefully place it in the pan. Press each spoonful down a little to flatten and continue until you have used up all your mixture (you should end up with about 12 small patties). Fry (in batches if necessary) for 5 minutes on one side, and when the bottom of the patties are golden brown flip them over gently using a palette knife or spatula and brown them on the other side. The falafel patties are ready when they are brown on both sides and hot in the middle. Remove them from the pan and transfer them to a plate lined with kitchen paper to soak up any excess oil.

Meanwhile, make the sweet chilli sauce. Put the honey and chilli in a small pan over a low heat and simmer for 3 minutes, stirring often. Pour the sauce into a small ramekin.

Warm the tortillas through in a dry pan over a low heat.

To serve:

4 seeded tortilla wraps or corn tortillas

4 tbsp cream cheese

Large handful of rocket

To assemble the wraps, spread a tablespoon of cream cheese over a warm tortilla, add a handful of rocket, some sweet chilli sauce and a few falafel patties. Repeat with the remaining wraps, cream cheese, rocket, chilli sauce and patties. Roll up and enjoy.

Tip:

If you are lactose intolerant, there are various alternatives to the cream cheese available, including soya and oat varieties.

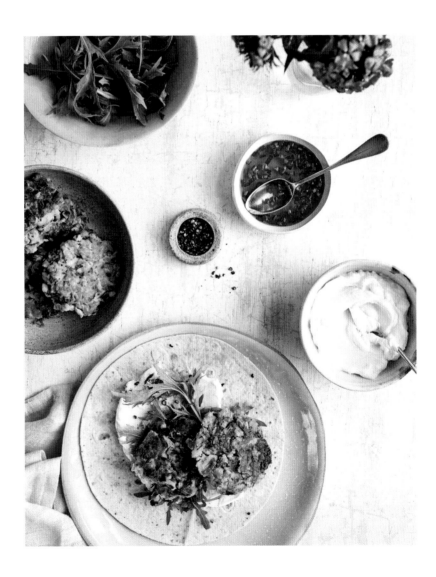

PEA, EDAMAME AND MINT FRITTATA

SERVES 1

This is one of my go-to lunches when I'm in a rush and it's great for taking to work. It takes under ten minutes to make, and has only a few ingredients, but is a good source of protein. Adding some feta is also delicious and, if you have more time and would like to add spring onions or asparagus (which take longer to cook), go ahead.

1 tbsp olive oil

50g frozen edamame beans

50g frozen petits pois

4 mint leaves, chopped

1 garlic clove, crushed

3 eggs

Splash of milk

Salt and freshly ground black pepper

Heat the oil in a large frying pan over a high heat. Add the edamame and peas to the pan and fry until warmed through, then add the mint and garlic and reduce the heat to medium.

Whisk the eggs in a mug with the milk and a pinch each of salt and pepper.

Spread the edamame and peas out evenly in the frying pan and pour over the eggs (the frittata will be thin, not thick). Cook for 5–8 minutes, until the eggs are cooked through, and serve hot or leave to cool.

Tip:

This frittata will be thin and will therefore cook quickly. If you would like to double the quantities to serve two, the frittata will take an extra 5 minutes to cook through.

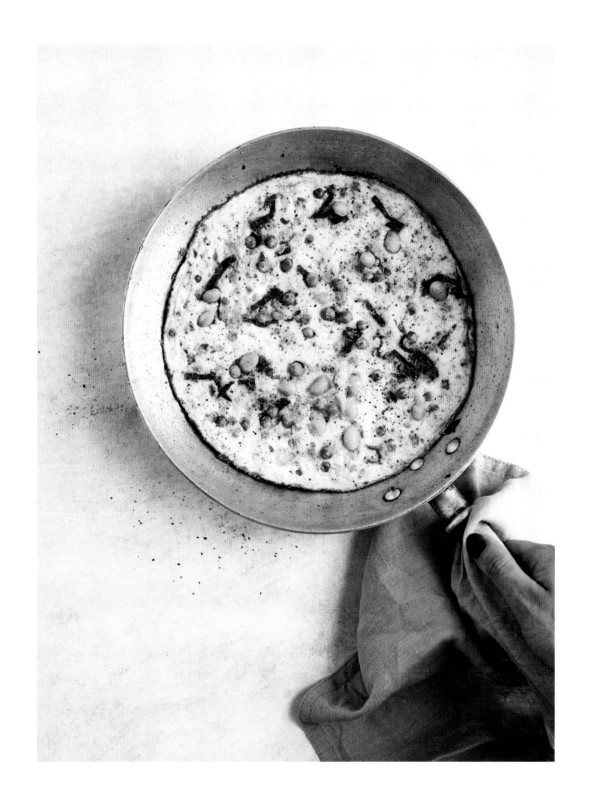

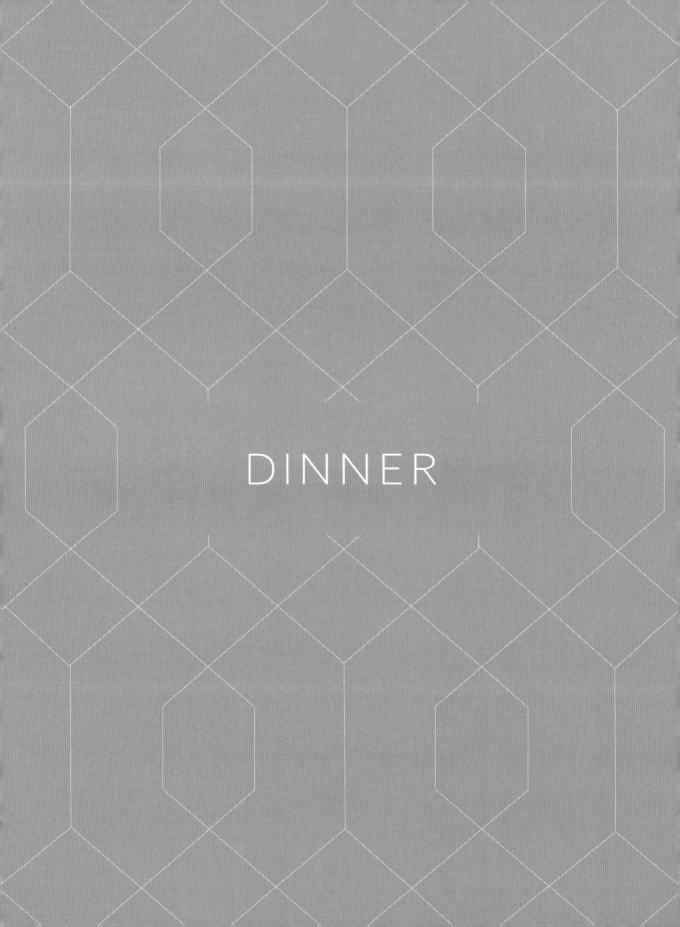

DINNER

INDIAN SPICED OAT FRIED CHICKEN
with Chilli and Coriander Corn

SERVES 2

Fried chicken is undeniably delicious, but it's also very high in the saturated fats it is fried in. The coating usually absorbs a lot of unhealthy fats and while the occasional piece might not kill you, this version is lower in fat. The chicken is roasted, rather than fried, and the oats provide fibre while the chicken provides protein.

For the chilli and coriander corn:

2 corn on the cobs

½ fresh red chilli, finely chopped

1 garlic clove, crushed

Small handful of fresh coriander, chopped

2 tsp butter

For the spiced fried chicken:

75g porridge oats

25g cashews

25g pumpkin seeds

1 tsp curry powder

½ tsp ground cumin

½ tsp turmeric

½ tsp ground coriander

1 egg

50g plain flour (or gluten-free flour)

2 skinless chicken breasts, cut into 2.5cm thick strips

1 tbsp olive oil

Sea salt and freshly ground black pepper

Preheat the oven to 180°C Fan (200°C/400°F/Gas Mark 6).

Cut or tear off two large squares of foil and lay them on your work surface. Add a corn cob to each, then divide the chilli, garlic and coriander between them, before topping each cob with a teaspoon of butter. Wrap the foil around the corn cobs and close the parcels tightly so no heat can escape. Put the foil parcels on a baking tray and pop it onto the top shelf of the oven for 30–35 minutes.

While the corn is in the oven, prepare the ingredients for the fried chicken. Put the oats, cashews, seeds, spices, coriander and a pinch of salt and pepper in a blender or food processor and blitz until the mixture resembles breadcrumbs (try not to over-blend – you don't want it to turn to dust).

Whisk the egg in a shallow bowl, tip the flour onto a plate and tip the spiced oat mix onto another plate.

Take each strip of chicken and coat it in the flour, then dip it in the egg and, finally, coat it evenly in the oat mixture. Lay the coated strips on a non-stick roasting tray, making sure they don't overlap. The chicken strips should have plenty of room on the tray – if not, divide them between two roasting trays.

Drizzle the coated chicken strips with the olive oil and place them in the oven when the corn has only 15 minutes left to cook, very carefully turning the chicken pieces over halfway through.

Serve the chicken with the corn, the chilli and coriander butter from the corn parcels and as many greens as you can fit on your plate.

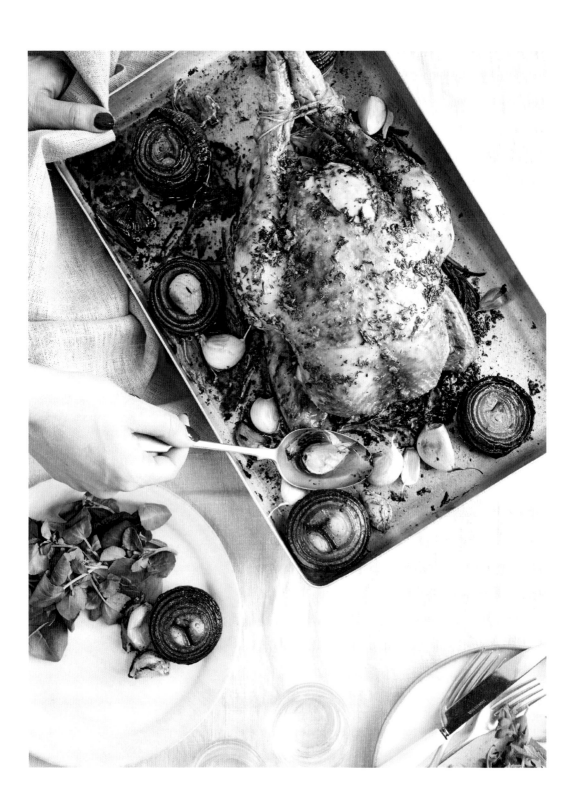

ROAST CHICKEN
with Rosemary, Garlic and Butter Marinade

SERVES 3–4

Almost every Sunday I cook a large roast chicken and it creates two or three incredible meals for the week. I try to buy the best chicken I can afford (remember, you are effectively eating what the chicken has eaten), as I will use absolutely all of it. Roasting the chicken with butter underneath the skin allows the herbs to flavour the meat and keeps the chicken moist.

1 large chicken (approx. 1.8kg, best quality, ideally organic)

150g good-quality butter, softened

7 rosemary sprigs, 3 with leaves picked and chopped, 4 left whole

9 large garlic cloves, 1 crushed and 8 left whole (skins on)

3 red onions, peeled and halved widthways

Sea salt and freshly ground black pepper

Preheat the oven to 180°C Fan (200°C/400°F/Gas Mark 6).

Find the neck end of the chicken and, using your fingers, gently pull the skin away from the breasts until you have created two pockets of space for the flavoured butter.

Put the butter, chopped rosemary, crushed garlic, and a pinch of salt and pepper in a bowl, and, using your hands, massage them together to create a paste.

Take a third of the butter and it put under the skin of one breast. Using your hands, start to massage the skin to disperse the butter, until you can see through the skin that it has spread throughout the pocket. Do the same with the other breast and spread the last third of the herby butter over the outside of the chicken, especially the legs.

Place the chicken in a roasting tray, put the onion halves cut-side down around the chicken and throw in the rosemary sprigs and whole garlic cloves.

Cook in the oven for 1 hour and 40 minutes, basting the chicken with its cooking juices every 30 minutes.

Remove the chicken from the oven and leave to rest for 10–15 minutes.

Serve the roast chicken with your favourite veg (for inspiration, see the Sides section on pages 92–99), a complex carb such as sweet potatoes, the whole roasted onions and the soft garlic squeezed out of its skin.

SQUASH AND LEEK GRATIN
with Sourdough and Parmesan Crumb

SERVES 2 AS
A MAIN OR
4 AS A SIDE

This gratin is one of my favourite recipes. It's warming and satisfying and the textures are amazing. I often see people throwing squash seeds away but they are so tasty and are full of amazing minerals. I like to serve this gratin on its own, but it's equally delicious as a side for a roast. Squash is a good source of vitamin A.

2 tsp coconut oil

2 leeks, washed and thickly sliced

1 large butternut squash, peeled and cut into 2cm cubes (seeds reserved)

2 garlic cloves, thinly sliced

6 thyme sprigs, leaves picked

1 tsp olive oil

Pinch of dried chilli flakes

300ml double cream

1 large slice of sourdough (or gluten-free bread)

15g Parmesan, grated

50g pine nuts

Sea salt and freshly ground black pepper

Preheat the oven to 180°C Fan (200°C/400°F/Gas Mark 6) and line a baking tray with baking parchment.

Melt the oil in a large frying pan over a medium heat, add the leeks and fry for 4 minutes until soft. Add the squash cubes, garlic, thyme and a pinch of salt and pepper and fry for 2 minutes, then tip everything into a large casserole dish and spread out evenly. Place the dish in the middle of the oven to roast for 20 minutes.

Meanwhile, rinse the reserved squash seeds, removing any of the stringy membrane that's still attached, and pat them dry with kitchen paper. Put them in a bowl and add the oil, salt and pepper and chilli flakes. Stir, then spread out evenly on the lined baking tray. Pop the tray onto the top rack of the oven to toast for around 5 minutes, shaking them halfway through. Keep a close eye on them as they can catch and burn easily. Remove and set to one side once toasted.

Remove the squash from the oven, pour the cream evenly over it and put it back in the oven for a further 20 minutes.

Meanwhile, blitz the bread in a food processor until it resembles fine breadcrumbs (or chop it finely by hand).

Remove the gratin from the oven and sprinkle it with the crumbs, Parmesan, pine nuts and a final pinch of black pepper and put it back in the oven for 5 minutes until golden brown on top. Serve with the toasted squash seeds sprinkled on top.

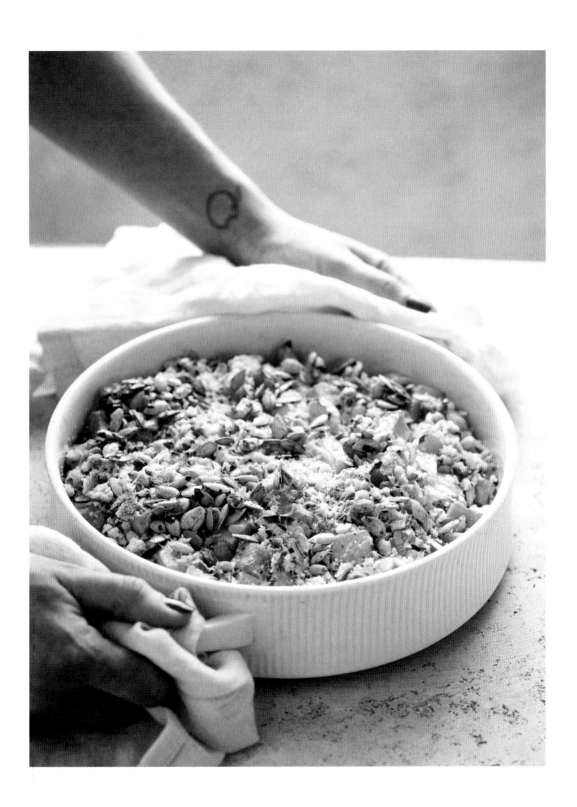

SPELTSOTTO
with King Prawns, Lemon and Thyme

SERVES 2

Risotto is one of my absolute favourite foods. I love the creamy texture, the slightly al dente bite of the rice and the fact that, except for all the stirring, it's pretty easy to cook. Quick-cook spelt makes it even easier, and much quicker to make. You only need to stir it occasionally, and it'll be ready within 20 minutes. Plus, spelt has more fibre than rice, which can help keep blood sugar levels stable, and prawns are high in protein.

Knob of butter or
1 tbsp of olive oil

2 leeks, washed
and sliced

2 garlic cloves,
crushed

6 thyme sprigs,
leaves picked

200g quick-cook
spelt

Splash of white wine
(optional)

500ml chicken (or
vegetable) stock

Grated zest and juice
of ½ lemon

160g raw shelled
king prawns

40g Parmesan, grated

Sprinkle of toasted
pine nuts

Small handful
of rocket

Good-quality
extra-virgin olive oil
(optional)

Place a large saucepan over a medium heat and add the butter (or oil) and leeks. Fry for about 5 minutes until the leeks are soft, then add the garlic, thyme and spelt. Fry for a further 2 minutes, then add the white wine, if using, and simmer for about 5 minutes (or until you can no longer smell the alcohol).

Add the stock, lemon zest and juice and simmer, stirring occasionally, for 10 minutes (until the spelt is cooked but still al dente), then add the prawns and Parmesan, stir, and cook for a further 2 minutes, until the prawns are pink and hot throughout.

Divide the mixture between two large bowls and top with the pine nuts, rocket and a drizzle of olive oil, if you wish.

Tip:
If you are vegan you could swap the prawns for roasted asparagus and leave out the Parmesan.

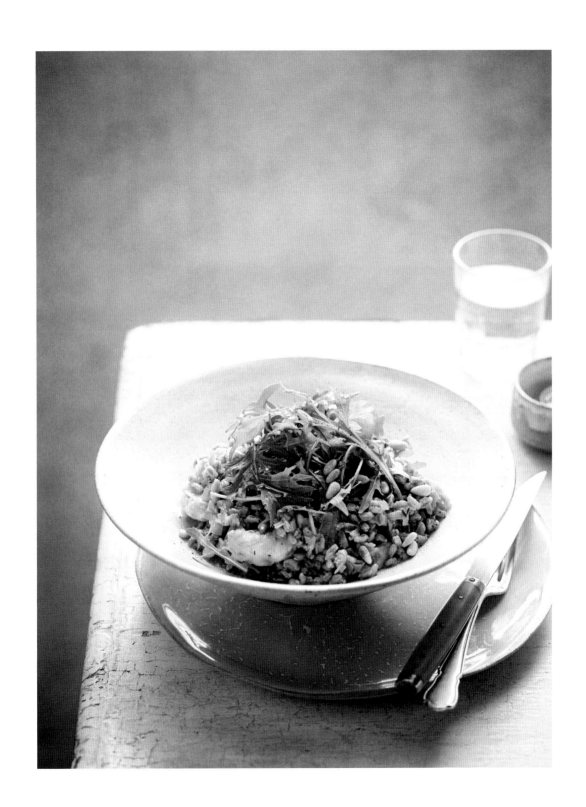

CHILLI AND SESAME TUNA POKE BOWL

SERVES 4

Poke bowls are a sort of deconstructed (and far easier) version of sushi. They are really simple to make and the recipe is very flexible, so feel free to swap in your favourite vegetables or fish. I serve the fish raw (which is incredible and smooth) but you could sauté it if you prefer. It's recommended we eat three portions of fish each week, one of which should be oily – this counts as one portion of oily fish.

For the tuna:

4 sushi-grade tuna steaks

½ fresh red chilli, finely chopped

2 tsp sriracha sauce

3 tbsp soy sauce

1 tbsp sesame oil

Small handful of fresh coriander, chopped

For the sushi rice:

400g sushi rice

520ml cold water

4 tbsp rice vinegar

4 tsp caster sugar

2 tsp fine salt

To serve:

6 spring onions, thinly sliced

1½ ripe avocados, peeled, stoned and thinly sliced

2 small carrots, grated

1 tbsp sesame seeds

Juice of 1 lime

Cut the tuna into small cubes and place them in a large bowl. Add the rest of the tuna ingredients, cover the bowl with cling film and leave it in the fridge for 30 minutes.

Meanwhile, cook the rice. Put the rice in a large bowl and cover it with cold water. Pass it through a sieve and repeat twice more. Put the rinsed rice in a large saucepan, add the cold water and cover with a lid. Bring to the boil, then reduce to a simmer and cook for 10 minutes. Take the pan off the heat (but keep the lid on) and leave for 10–15 minutes to steam.

In a separate medium bowl combine the vinegar, sugar and salt. Add the cooked rice to the bowl, gently folding it through the vinegar marinade.

Divide the sushi rice between four bowls, top with the tuna, then add the spring onions, avocado and grated carrot. Top with the sesame seeds, drizzle with lime juice and serve.

Tips:

Ensure you ask for sushi-grade fish from your fishmonger or shop if you are planning on eating the fish raw, and make sure it is as fresh as possible.

For a vegetarian poke bowl, leave out the fish and supplement it with extra vegetables or marinated tofu.

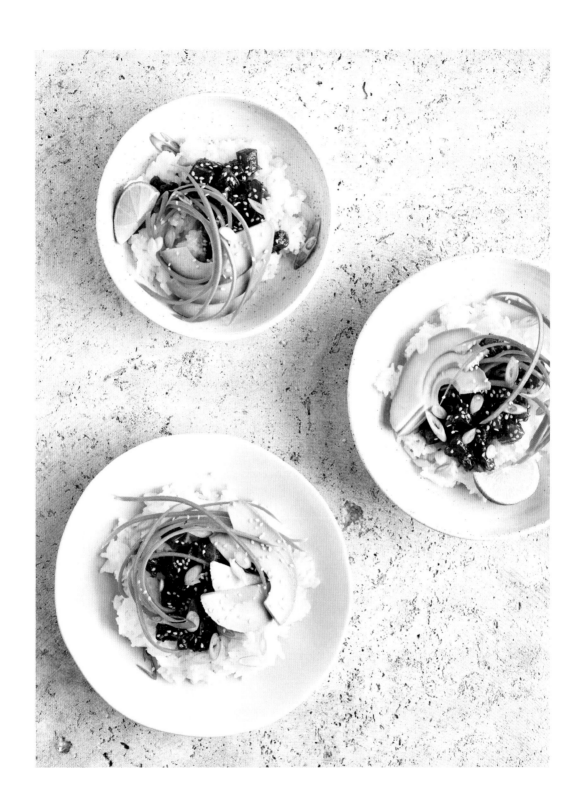

SALMON, LEMONGRASS AND GINGER PATTIES

SERVES 2

Fishcakes are delicious but can be time-consuming to make when potato is involved. These salmon patties have no potato, so are quick to prepare and are a good source of protein. They also count as one of your portions of oily fish. They are delicious with sweet potato wedges and Soy, Sesame and Honey-glazed Carrots (page 95).

2 fresh salmon fillets

1cm piece of fresh root ginger, peeled and grated

1cm piece of lemongrass, finely chopped

1 garlic clove, crushed

2 spring onions, thinly sliced

1 egg yolk

Small handful of fresh coriander, chopped

1 tbsp coconut oil

Sea salt and freshly ground black pepper

Using a sharp knife, carefully cut the skin away from the salmon fillets, then cut the salmon into very small cubes. Put the salmon in a large bowl and add all the remaining ingredients (except the oil), season with salt and pepper, mix together and leave to rest for 5 minutes.

Heat the oil in a large frying pan over a high heat. Scoop up a tablespoonful of the salmon mixture and carefully place it in the hot pan. Continue scooping up the rest of the mixture and placing it in the pan (you should have enough mixture to make about 6 patties in total), using the back of the spoon to carefully press the patties down so they bind together (treat them gently).

Fry for 4–5 minutes until brown underneath, then carefully flip and cook for a further 4–5 minutes until cooked through. Transfer to a plate lined with kitchen paper to absorb any excess oil, and serve.

WHOLEWHEAT SPAGHETTI
with Caramelised Sprouts, Lemon and Garlic

SERVES 2

I love pasta, and wholewheat spaghetti has a higher fibre content than regular spaghetti. I also find it has a better texture for this recipe. Sprouts are delicious when cooked in butter until brown, and the lemon cuts through their earthiness. This is genuinely one of my favourite go-to lunches (as you may have seen from my social media). This recipe is also a source of protein, as well as fibre.

160g wholewheat spaghetti (organic if possible)

1 tbsp butter

1 tbsp olive oil

1 red onion, thinly sliced

1 rosemary sprig, leaves picked and chopped

Small pinch of dried chilli flakes

150g Brussels sprouts, thinly sliced

2 garlic cloves, thinly sliced

Grated zest and juice of ½ lemon

Small handful of grated Parmesan (optional)

Small handful of toasted pine nuts (optional)

Sea salt

Bring a large saucepan of salted water to the boil, add the spaghetti and cook according to the packet instructions, until al dente.

Meanwhile, heat the butter and oil in a large frying pan over a high heat and add the onion, rosemary, chilli flakes and sprouts. Fry for about 10 minutes, stirring frequently to prevent burning, until the sprouts are lightly browned. Add the garlic and lemon zest with a good pinch of salt, fry for a further 2 minutes, then remove from the heat.

Drain the pasta, reserving 2 tablespoons of the cooking water. Add the pasta to the frying pan with the reserved pasta cooking water and the sprouts, and mix to combine. Add the Parmesan, if using, and stir.

Divide the pasta between two bowls and serve, topped with pine nuts, if using, and a drizzle of the lemon juice.

Tip:

There are plenty of great gluten-free pastas available now. Many are even stocked in larger supermarkets. You can also swap the spaghetti for your favourite vegetable alternative such as squash or courgette noodles.

STEAK AND BLACK BEAN BURRITOS
with Coriander Guacamole

SERVES 2

This burrito recipe can be adapted in so many ways: lean red meat is a great source of protein and iron, but if you don't eat meat, strips of marinated tofu are delicious instead of the steak; and you can also swap the black beans for tinned kidney beans or lentils. Corn tortillas have more fibre and less saturated fats than wheat flour tortillas – try to buy the best quality you can, as many contain added flour (corn tortillas are usually just made of cornmeal, oil and water). The black beans can be made a day ahead.

STEAK COOKING TIMES:

Rare: 1 ½ minutes on each side

Medium: 2½ minutes on each side

Medium rare: 2 minutes on each side

Well done: 4–5 minutes on each side

2 small sirloin steaks

1 tsp olive oil

Pinch of dried chilli flakes

2 large or 4 small corn tortillas

Large handful of rocket

Sea salt and freshly ground black pepper

For the spiced black beans:

1 tsp olive oil

½ red onion, finely chopped

½ fresh red chilli, finely chopped

½ yellow pepper, chopped

1 garlic clove, chopped

To make the spiced black beans, heat the oil in a medium saucepan over a medium heat, add the onion, red chilli, yellow pepper and garlic and fry for 5 minutes. When the onions are soft but not browned, add the beans, spices, and coriander, stir, cover and leave over a low heat to stay warm.

Mash the avocado in a bowl then add the coriander, spring onions, lime juice and some black pepper to taste. Cover the bowl with cling film and set aside.

Heat a large frying pan over a high heat until smoking hot. Rub the steaks with a little oil and season with a little sea salt, pepper and the chilli flakes then lay them carefully in the hot pan. Cook the steaks using the guidelines above, based on how well done you like them, then transfer them to a warm plate and leave at room temperature to rest for 4–5 minutes.

Warm through the tortillas in a dry pan over a low heat.

Lay the tortillas onto plates, divide the rocket, beans and guacamole between them, then slice the rested steaks and place on top. Fold up carefully and enjoy.

200g tinned black
beans, drained
and rinsed

½ tsp hot paprika

½ tsp ground cumin

½ tsp ground
coriander

**For the coriander
guacamole:**

$^2/_3$ ripe avocado

Small handful of fresh
coriander, chopped

3 spring onions,
thinly sliced

Juice of ½ lime

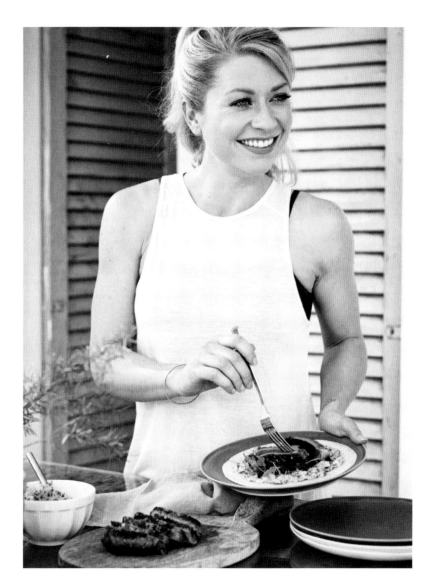

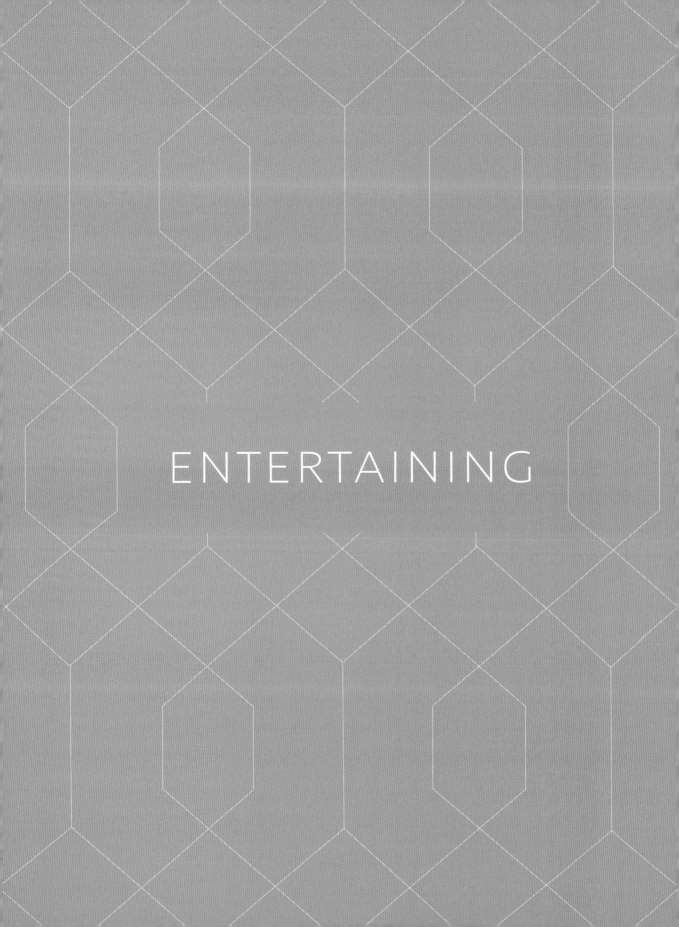

ENTERTAINING

SQUASH AND ROSEMARY CARBONARA

SERVES 4

Friday night in our house means pizza for my husband and pasta for me. I love pasta — always have and always will — and hate the bad press it receives. If you are gluten intolerant there are some amazing alternatives out there, such as brown rice pasta or courgetti, and if you aren't intolerant, pasta should be enjoyed guilt-free as part of a balanced diet. This recipe is comforting, creamy and addictive!

1 squash (butternut or crown prince works best), halved, deseeded, peeled and cut into 2cm cubes

Pinch of dried chilli flakes

4 rosemary sprigs, rinsed

1½ tbsp olive oil

2 red onions, diced

4 garlic cloves, crushed

250g fresh tagliatelle

300ml single cream

2 whole eggs, plus 2 egg yolks

50g Parmesan, grated

10 walnuts, broken up

Sea salt and freshly ground black pepper

Preheat the oven to 180°C Fan (200°C/400°F/Gas Mark 6).

Put the cubes of squash in a large roasting tray with the chilli flakes, rosemary sprigs and ½ tablespoon of the oil, season with salt and pepper, toss to coat and pop the tray in the oven for 20–30 minutes, stirring occasionally to prevent the squash catching on the bottom of the tray. You want it to brown only slightly and be soft throughout, so turn down the oven by 10°C if they are getting crispy.

Heat the rest of the oil in your largest frying pan over a medium heat, add the onions and fry for about 10 minutes until caramelised then add the garlic and fry for a further minute. Add the cooked squash (with some of the rosemary leaves from the stalks) and reduce the heat to low to keep the squash warm.

Bring a large saucepan of salted water to the boil, add the pasta and cook it according to the packet instructions (this should take about 3–5 minutes). While the pasta is cooking, whisk the cream, eggs and grated Parmesan in a jug. Once the pasta is cooked, drain it, reserving 2 tablespoons of the cooking water, and pour it all back into the saucepan (off the heat).

Add the squash, onions, cream and egg mix and stir. Divide between four plates and top with the broken walnuts.

Tip:

I spent years draining my pasta to death only to have to add copious amounts of olive oil to stop it being dry. Reserving some of your pasta cooking water helps to prevent the pasta drying out too much and helps to loosen your sauce.

CASHEW AND OAT PANCAKES
with Sautéed Peaches, Orange Yoghurt and Bacon

SERVES 4
(MAKES 12
PANCAKES)

This quick dish is ideal for a weekend brunch. The pancakes are really filling and high in fibre and protein, and the sautéed peaches are soft and sweet. You can swap the peaches for nectarines, mango or plums. I like to make the bacon extra crispy to add texture to the dish, and I love sweet and salty flavours together, but feel free to leave it out.

2 small knobs
of butter

2 peaches, halved,
stones removed and
flesh cut into 2.5cm-
thick slices

1 tsp honey

4 rashers of good-
quality unsmoked
streaky bacon

160g porridge oats

160g cashews

2 large bananas,
peeled and chopped

4 eggs

Splash of milk

Grated zest of
1 orange

4 tbsp Greek
yoghurt

Preheat the grill.

Melt one knob of butter in a large frying pan over a medium heat then add the peach slices and honey. Fry for 5–6 minutes until golden and caramelised on each side, watching them carefully to make sure they don't burn.

Place the bacon rashers on a grill pan under the hot grill, turning them occasionally until crisp. Meanwhile, put the oats, cashews, bananas, eggs and milk in a blender and blitz until you have a smooth batter.

When the pancakes are cooked on both sides, stir the zest into the yoghurt (don't do this ahead of time, as it will make the yoghurt watery).

Stack the pancakes on plates, add a dollop of yoghurt to each stack, along with the peaches, and top with the crisp bacon rashers.

Tip:

If cooking the pancakes in two batches, pop the first batch into a low oven to keep warm until they are all ready.

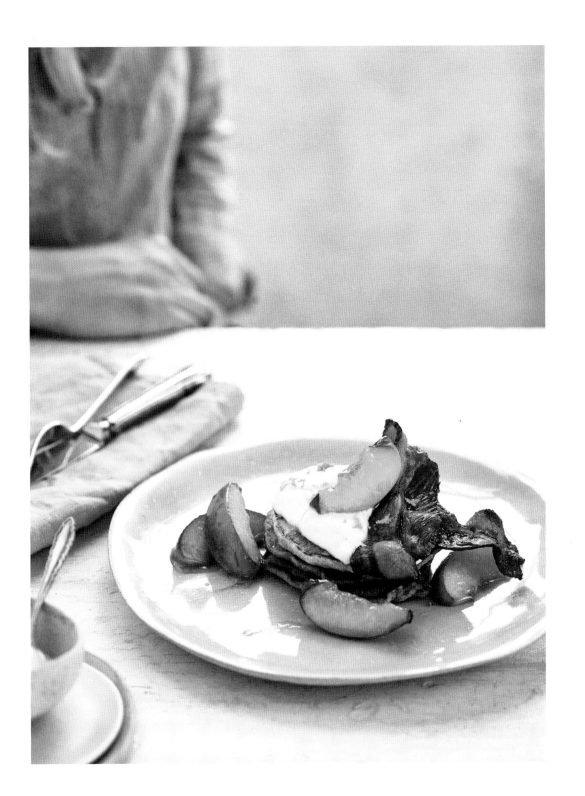

LENTIL DAL, SPICED ROAST CAULIFLOWER AND MINT YOGHURT

SERVES 3

I love Indian food, and the more fragrant it is, the better. This dal has a few components but they are all well worth the effort. I love serving this on a large platter so people can help themselves to the accompaniments. Lentils are an incredible source of fibre, which helps to maintain a healthy digestive system. This recipe also contributes two portions of vegetables to your five-a-day and is a high source of fibre and a source of protein. The mint yoghurt cuts through the spices of the dal beautifully.

For the dal:

350g red split lentils, rinsed

1 litre good-quality vegetable stock (low-salt if possible)

2 tsp turmeric

1 tbsp olive oil

2 tsp curry powder or garam masala

½ tsp cumin seeds, crushed

½ tsp fennel seeds, crushed

½ tsp coriander seeds, crushed

½ fresh red chilli, thinly sliced

1 large red onion, thinly sliced

4 garlic cloves, finely chopped

2 large carrots, grated

Preheat the oven to 160°C Fan (180°C/350°F/Gas Mark 4).

Rinse the lentils and place them in a large saucepan with the stock and turmeric. Bring to the boil, then lower the heat and simmer for 25–30 minutes, or until the lentils are soft.

Meanwhile, spread the cauliflower florets out in a large roasting tray. Drizzle over the oil, then add a generous grind of fresh black pepper and the curry powder or garam masala. Toss to coat and pop the tray in the oven for 20 minutes, turning the cauliflower florets halfway through.

When the lentils are almost done, heat the oil in a large frying pan over a medium heat, add the spices, fennel, coriander and chilli and fry for 2 minutes until fragrant. Add the onion, garlic and carrots and fry for 5–6 minutes until soft, then reduce the heat to low.

Mix the ingredients for the yoghurt together in a bowl and leave to one side.

When the lentils are soft, add them to the onion and carrot mixture in the pan. Stir well, adding a little more pepper if needed. Divide between four bowls, and serve with the roasted cauliflower (sprinkle a little extra curry powder or garam masala on top, if you like) and mint yoghurt dressing on the side, for people to help themselves.

For the roasted cauliflower:

400g cauliflower, broken into mini florets

2 tbsp olive oil

2 tsp curry powder or garam masala, plus extra to serve

Freshly ground black pepper

For the mint yoghurt:

4 tbsp Greek yoghurt

Large handful of fresh mint, chopped

Juice of ½ lemon

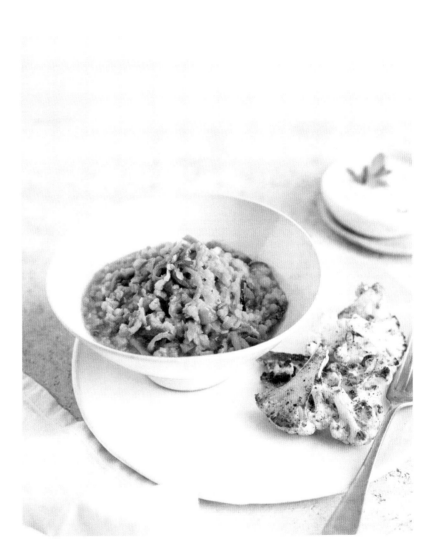

Tip:

You can swap the red lentils for any you have in your cupboard (the recipe also works well with green lentils) and use non-dairy alternatives for the yoghurt, if you prefer.

BEETROOT, FENNEL, THYME AND GOATS' CHEESE TART

SERVES 4–6

Beetroot is so delicious roasted, but can take a long time to cook. In this recipe, the grated beetroot takes only 15 minutes to become soft and delicious and the goats' cheese cuts through its earthy flavours. This is a great centrepiece for a dinner party or can be made into individual tarts if you prefer. It is also a source of protein.

375g pack of ready-rolled all-butter puff pastry

2 beetroots, washed

1 fennel bulb, washed

1 red onion, peeled

8 thyme sprigs, leaves picked

75g goats' cheese, crumbled

1 tbsp olive oil

Splash of milk

To serve:

Large handful of rocket

1 tbsp balsamic vinegar

Small handful of shaved Parmesan

Sea salt and freshly ground black pepper

Preheat the oven to 180°C Fan (200°C/400°F/Gas Mark 6).

Unroll the pastry onto a large, flat baking sheet and place it in the fridge.

Grate the beetroot, fennel and onion into a large mixing bowl and stir in the thyme, goats' cheese and oil. Season with salt and pepper.

Take the pastry out of the fridge and, using a sharp knife, score a border around the edge of the pastry, about 2.5cm in from the edge. Brush the edge with the milk using a pastry brush.

Pour the beetroot, fennel and onion filling into the middle of the pastry, within the border, and gently spread it out to meet the scored line. Bake in the oven for 15–20 minutes, until the pastry is golden brown.

Serve warm, topped with the rocket, drizzled with the balsamic vinegar and sprinkled with the Parmesan shavings.

Tips:

Beetroot stains, so wear rubber gloves when you grate it, and don't use your favourite chopping board. Try to keep all the beetroot in the bowl (not on your work surfaces).

My husband doesn't like fennel, so if he's eating this dish, I don't use it, and it works just as well – add an extra beetroot if you're leaving it out.

LAMB, CHICKPEA AND APRICOT TAGINE

SERVES 4

This is one of my absolute favourite recipes. Cooking the lamb low and slow creates the most tender meat. The spices are warming and fragrant and the almonds and pomegranate seeds add texture to the dish. It is a good source of protein and fibre. Serve with quinoa or brown rice (ideally cooked in vegetable stock). It tastes even better reheated the next day.

2 tsp coconut oil or butter

500g diced lamb

2 red onions, diced

1 carrot, peeled and diced

2 garlic cloves, crushed

3cm piece of fresh root ginger, peeled and grated

1½ tsp hot paprika

1 tsp ground cinnamon

1½ tsp ground cumin

2 cloves, crushed

1 tsp fennel seeds

400g tin of chickpeas, drained and rinsed

400g tin of chopped tomatoes

100g dried apricots, quartered

Juice of ½ lemon

400ml lamb stock

Large handful of fresh coriander, chopped

Sea salt and freshly ground black pepper

To serve:

80g pomegranate seeds

100g flaked almonds

Grated zest of 1 lemon

Preheat the oven to 160°C Fan (180°C/350°F/Gas Mark 4).

Melt the oil or butter in a large ovenproof casserole dish over a high heat. Add the lamb and fry for 5–6 minutes until lightly browned (in batches if necessary), then scoop the lamb out and set aside in a dish.

Reduce the heat to medium and add the onions, carrot, garlic, ginger, spices and fennel to the casserole dish. Fry, stirring constantly, for 4–5 minutes until the onions are soft (watch the garlic doesn't burn) then add the lamb back to the dish. Increase the heat slightly, tip in the rest of the ingredients, except the coriander, and season with salt and pepper. Bring to the boil, pop on the lid and place in the middle of the oven for 1 hour 30 minutes, stirring it every 30 minutes. Remove the dish from the oven and let it rest for 5 minutes before serving.

Stir through the chopped coriander, serve with Apricot, Mint and Pistachio Quinoa (page 98) and top each serving with the pomegranate seeds, flaked almonds and lemon zest.

Tip:

If you are vegan, replace the lamb with half a butternut squash, cubed, and swap the lamb stock for vegetable stock.

ROAST CHICKEN THIGHS
with Lemon, Thyme and Garlic

SERVES 2

These chicken thighs take very little effort to cook. You simply assemble the ingredients and leave them to roast in the oven. The chicken should be juicy and tender, and the skin crispy. The lemon and garlic caramelises when it's baked and I love eating the garlic straight out of its skin. I like to serve this with my Green Beans with Crispy Shallots, Pine Nuts and Garlic (page 94) and a small roasted sweet potato which counts as two of your five-a-day.

4 chicken thighs, skin on and bone in

Small knob of butter

2 lemons, washed and quartered

4 thyme sprigs

8 garlic cloves, skin left on

Sea salt and freshly ground black pepper

Preheat the oven to 160°C Fan (180°C/350°F/Gas Mark 4).

Pat the skin of the chicken thighs dry with kitchen paper and season them generously with salt and pepper.

Melt the butter in a large frying pan over a high heat, place the thighs skin-side down in the frying pan and fry for about 5 minutes until the skin is browned and starting to crisp. Turn the thighs over and sear for 30 seconds on the other side, then transfer them to a small ovenproof dish skin-side up (you want them to sit neatly next to each other, not spaced out).

Tuck the lemon quarters, thyme and garlic into the gaps around the thighs and roast in the oven for 20–25 minutes. The thighs are ready when the meat is cooked through and piping hot throughout.

Tip:
Don't be afraid to slightly char the chicken skin in the frying pan – you want the skin to be crispy so the high heat is necessary. You may need a splatter guard over your pan as the fat can spit.

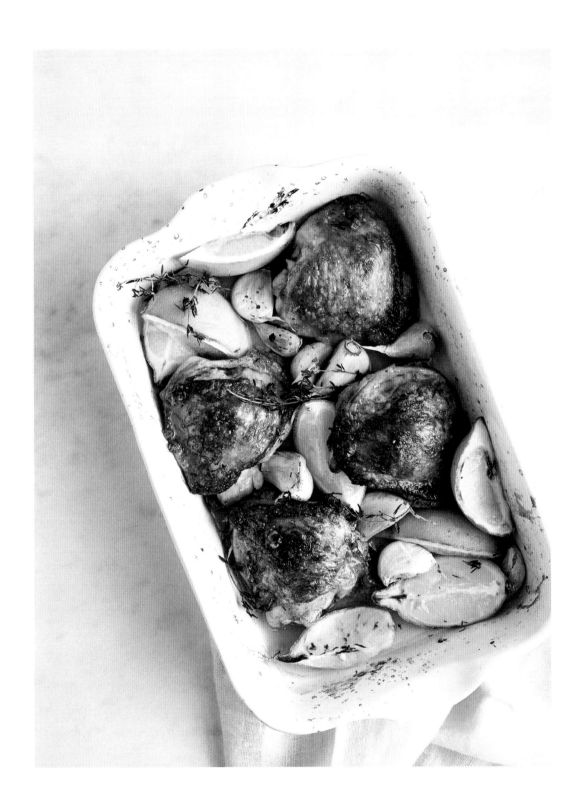

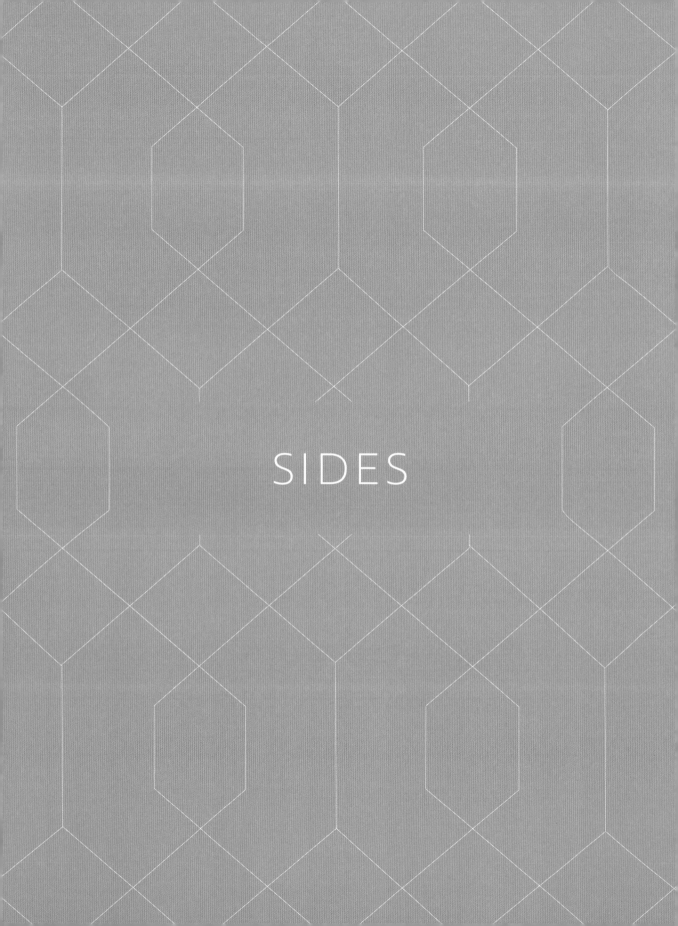

SIDES

AUBERGINE AND HARISSA HUMMUS

SERVES 4

Hummus is great for a mid-afternoon snack with crudités such as endive leaves, radishes, fennel or sugar snap peas. Harissa is a spicy North African chilli paste with rose, garlic and saffron. It adds heat to the hummus, and the roasted aubergine gives the hummus a wonderful silky texture. Tahini, made from ground sesame seeds, is high in unsaturated fats and calcium, and adds a nutty taste.

1 aubergine, washed

2 tbsp olive oil

400g tin of chickpeas, drained and rinsed

1 small garlic clove

2 tsp harissa paste

Juice of ½ lemon

1 tbsp tahini

Sea salt and freshly ground black pepper

Preheat the grill to medium (if you don't have a grill, use a hot oven instead).

Slice the aubergine in half lengthways. Holding each half on a board cut-side up, use a small, sharp knife to score the flesh in a criss-cross pattern (being careful not to cut the skin) and lay them on a grill pan or metal tray lined with foil. Rub the olive oil over the two halves with your hands and season them with salt and pepper. Place the aubergine under the grill for 10–15 minutes, until the flesh is soft throughout, turning the halves over if the flesh starts to burn.

Scrape the aubergine flesh into a food processor, add the rest of the ingredients and blitz to a smooth paste. Taste and season if needed.

Tip:

I love aubergines and often serve them grilled as in this recipe as a side dish. When doing so I grill on medium until soft, then turn the grill to high at the end so the flesh gets a little crispy and almost burnt.

GREEN BEANS
with Crispy Shallots, Pine Nuts and Garlic

SERVES 2

Green beans on their own can be a little bland, so I love adding crispy shallots, pine nuts and sautéing them in a little garlic. You can prove anyone who says they don't like vegetables wrong with this dish and it's an easy way to get in one of your five-a-day.

½ tbsp butter

4 shallots, thinly sliced

160g fine green beans, ends trimmed

1 garlic clove, thinly sliced

Small handful of toasted pine nuts

Sea salt

Melt the butter in a large frying pan over a high heat, add the shallots and fry for 5 minutes until they start to turn golden brown.

Steam the green beans in a steamer (or a colander over boiling water) for 4–5 minutes, or until al dente. Drain and immediately add them to the shallots in the pan, reducing the heat to medium. Add the garlic, pine nuts and a pinch of sea salt, mix well and serve.

SPICY THAI FRIED AUBERGINE

SERVES 2

The texture of aubergine often puts people off, but these are sticky and a little crispy so have a bit of bite.

1 tbsp olive oil

1 aubergine, cut into small chunks

$1/3$ fresh red chilli, finely chopped

2 tbsp soy sauce

2 tsp honey

1 tsp lime juice

1 tsp sesame oil

1 garlic clove, thinly sliced

Heat the olive oil in a large, non-stick frying pan over a high heat. Add the aubergine and chilli and stir-fry for around 5 minutes, until the aubergine begins to crisp up and brown. Add the soy sauce, honey, lime juice and sesame oil and stir-fry for a further 3–4 minutes until sticky and soft. Add the garlic and fry for a further minute then serve.

SOY, SESAME AND HONEY-GLAZED CARROTS

SERVES 2

These carrots are both sweet and salty (a taste sensation I love), and really simple to make. You could use a baby carrot such as Chantenay or cut the carrots into batons. I love serving these with the Roast Chicken on page 71.

500g carrots, scrubbed and cut into 2.5cm-thick batons

1 tbsp sunflower oil

1 tbsp low-sodium soy sauce

1 tbsp runny honey

2 tbsp sesame seeds

Sea salt and cracked black pepper

Preheat the oven to 180°C Fan (200°C/400°F/Gas Mark 6).

Put the carrot batons in a large roasting tin and coat with the oil. Season with salt and pepper and roast in the oven for 30 minutes, shaking the tray halfway through to ensure they cook evenly.

Add the soy sauce and honey to the roasting tin, toss, and continue to roast for a further 15 minutes, then add the sesame seeds, toss again, and roast for a final 5 minutes. Remove from the oven and serve.

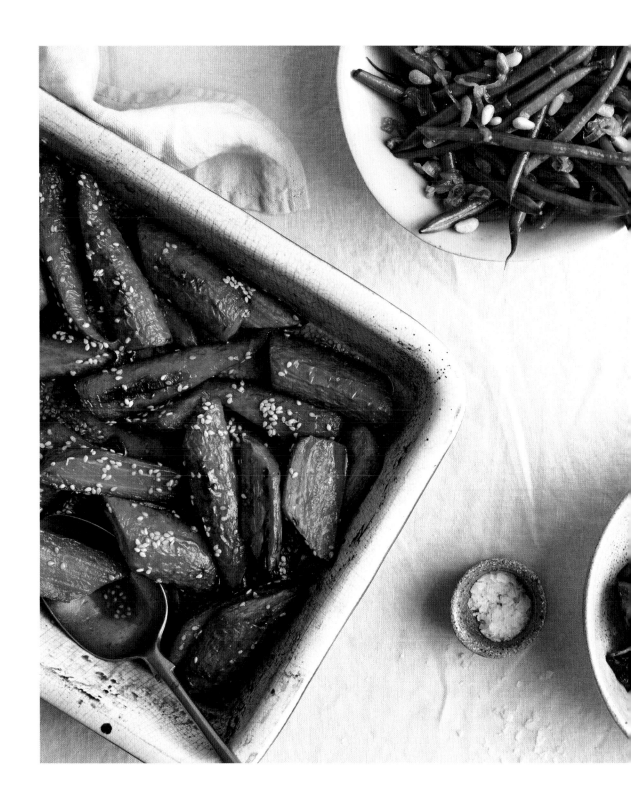

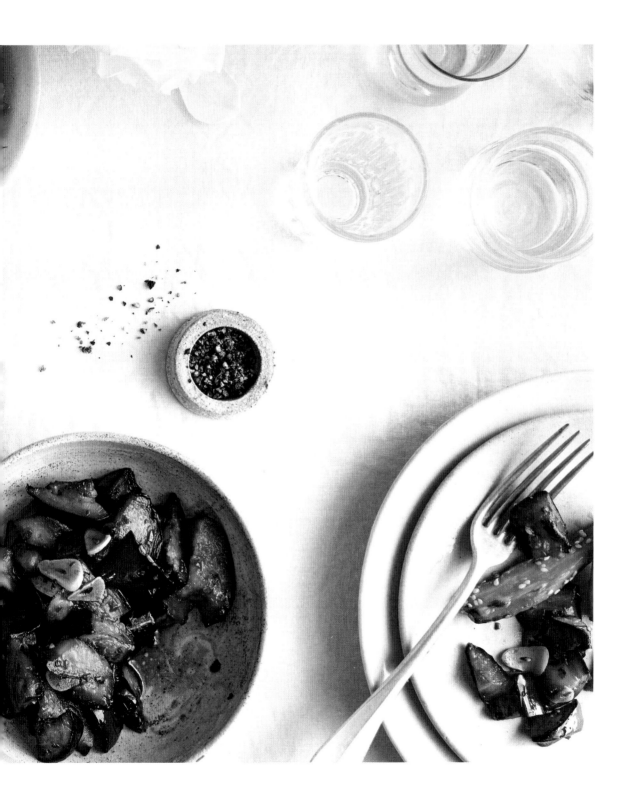

APRICOT, MINT AND PISTACHIO QUINOA

SERVES 2

This is a really fresh, easy quinoa recipe that is perfect in the Nourish Bowl (page 62) or as a side dish to any meal. Quinoa is a complete source of protein as it contains all nine essential amino acids, making it ideal for vegans. It is also high in fibre. You can dress up brown rice or spelt in the same way.

90g quinoa, rinsed

200ml hot vegetable stock (low-salt if possible)

4 dried apricots, roughly chopped

Small handful of pistachios, roughly chopped

Small handful of mint, roughly chopped

1 tsp flaxseed or rapeseed oil

Pinch of freshly cracked black pepper

Put the quinoa and stock in a medium saucepan and bring to the boil over a high heat. Reduce the heat and simmer for 10–15 minutes, until the quinoa is soft and the stock has been absorbed. If all the water is absorbed before the quinoa is cooked, add a little extra water. You want the quinoa to be dry by the time it's ready – you should not need to drain it.

Tip the quinoa into a medium bowl, add the rest of the ingredients and give it all a good stir. Season to taste (remember stock can contain a lot of salt so I wouldn't add any more).

BEETROOT, ORANGE AND POPPY SEED SALAD

SERVES 2

Beetroot is a good source of folate, which is needed to make DNA. Its earthy flavour is balanced with the tang of apple cider vinegar and the sweetness of orange. The poppy seeds add texture (sunflower seeds would also work well). I use this in my Nourish Bowl (see page 62) and it's also delicious with salmon. Use rubber gloves to handle the beetroot if possible, as it stains your hands easily.

2 beetroots, peeled and grated

Juice of ½ orange

1 tbsp apple cider vinegar

2 tbsp poppy seeds

Sea salt and freshly ground black pepper

Mix all ingredients together in a bowl and season to taste with salt and pepper.

Tip:

If you do stain your hands with beetroot, rubbing them with lemon juice will help get rid of the stains.

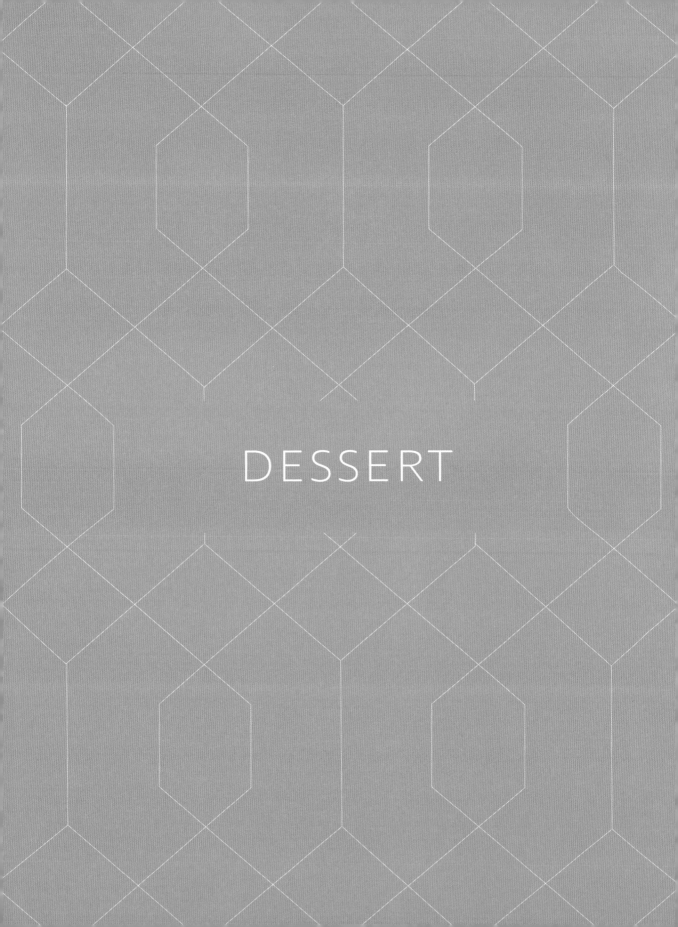

DESSERT

A CHOCOLATIER'S HOT CHOCOLATE

SERVES 1

When I was a chocolatier I used to absolutely love the hot chocolate we made (and probably drank more of it than I served – shh, don't tell anyone!). It was made with Amedei dark chocolate (which is simply incredible), whole milk and various other secret ingredients. Here is my take on it, with two flavour variations. Powdered hot chocolates can have a lot of added sugars or sweeteners, so I like that fact that there's very little messing around with ingredients here. All the spices are optional, so if you don't like chilli, simply leave it out. You can use your favourite milk here if you don't drink cow's milk. I've added the liquid ingredients in grams rather than millilitres to save you from washing up a measuring jug, but feel free to use grams, if you prefer!

Chai spiced hot chocolate:

250g semi-skimmed milk, or your favourite nut milk

Large pinch of ground cinnamon

Large pinch of turmeric

Large pinch of ground ginger

Small pinch of chilli powder

Couple gratings of nutmeg

40g dark chocolate (minimum 70% cocoa solids), finely chopped

For the chai spiced hot chocolate: Heat the milk and spices gently in a small saucepan, stirring throughout to prevent the milk catching at the bottom of the pan. Once the edges of the milk are just starting to bubble (don't let it come to a boil) remove the pan from the heat. Whisk in the chocolate until it has completely melted, taste and adjust the spices to taste, as you prefer. Pour the hot chocolate into a big mug, add a final grating of nutmeg and enjoy.

Orange and clove hot chocolate:

250g semi-skimmed milk, or your favourite nut milk

Seeds from ½ vanilla pod

Grated zest of ½ orange

2 whole cloves

40g dark chocolate (minimum 70% cocoa solids), finely chopped, plus extra to serve

For the orange and clove hot chocolate: Heat the milk, vanilla seeds, orange zest and cloves gently in a small saucepan, stirring throughout to prevent the milk catching at the bottom of the pan. Once the edges of the milk are just starting to bubble (don't let it come to a boil) remove the pan from the heat. Take out the cloves – you don't want to chew on those. Whisk in the chocolate until it has completely melted, taste and adjust the spices to taste, as you prefer. Pour the hot chocolate into a big mug, and add a final grating of chocolate and enjoy.

ROSEMARY AND CHOCOLATE BANANA BREAD

MAKES 6–8
SLICES

Bananas are like avocados – they often seem to be either too hard or too ripe. This recipe is a great way to use up overripe bananas, while rosemary and chocolate are a delicious combination. I use wholewheat flour and oats to add extra fibre to this gorgeous loaf.

100ml olive oil, plus extra for greasing

100g runny honey

3 very ripe small bananas, peeled

2 eggs

Seeds from ½ vanilla pod (pod retained)

2 tsp chopped fresh rosemary leaves

150g wholewheat flour

40g porridge oats

1 tsp baking powder

60g dark chocolate (minimum 70% cocoa solids), chopped

Preheat the oven to 160°C Fan (180°C/350°F/Gas Mark 4) and grease a 2lb loaf tin with oil. Line the tin with baking parchment on all sides, with enough overhanging to pull the baked cake out easily.

Add the oil, honey and bananas to a large mixing bowl and blend until smooth with an electric handheld whisk.

With the whisk still running, add the eggs, vanilla seeds (keep the pod for later) and rosemary to the mixture and blend until well combined.

In a separate bowl, combine the flour, oats, baking powder and chocolate. Tip the flour mixture into the banana mixture and slowly fold the flour mixture in, using a large metal spoon, until well combined.

Pour the batter into the prepared loaf tin, pop it into the middle of the oven and bake for 40–45 minutes, until a skewer inserted into the middle of the cake comes out clean.

After the cake has been baking for 30 minutes, cut the vanilla pod in half lengthways to give you two long, thin strips. Rest the strips on top of the banana bread and return it to the oven for the remaining 10–15 minutes.

Remove the banana bread from the oven and leave it to cool in the loaf tin for 10 minutes before gently running a knife around the edge of the loaf to loosen it. Turn it out carefully onto a wire rack to cool completely.

Tip:

I love adding herbs to desserts but please feel free to leave them out if it's not your cup of tea.

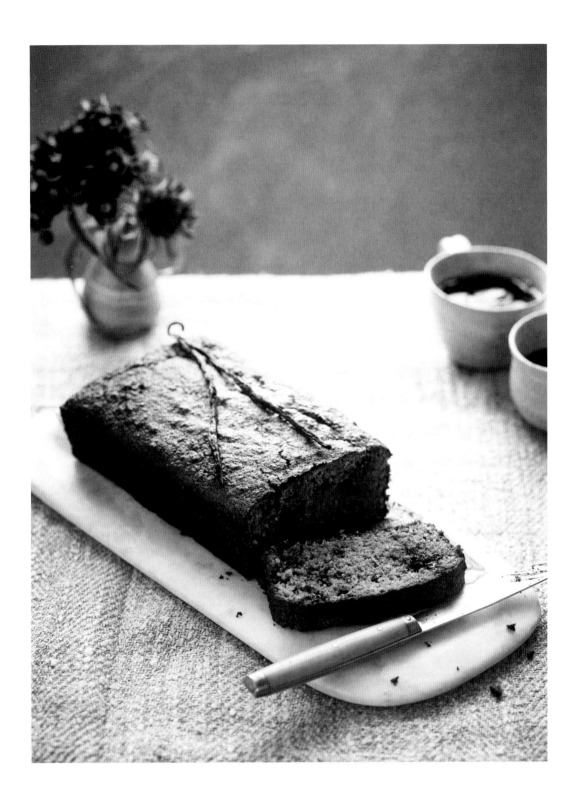

APPLE, APRICOT AND THYME CRUMBLE

SERVES 4–6

I absolutely love crumbles, and they are a great way to use up whatever fruit is in season, especially if you grow your own and have a glut. I have used dried apricots in this crumble to reduce the amount of free sugars needed in the recipe, and the oats, seeds and wholewheat flour all add extra fibre to the dish. The smell of the thyme is incredible while the flavour is quite subtle. Adding herbs to desserts adds an extra level of flavour and I find it stops people simply gobbling it down – they take their time and listen out for the flavours.

For the base:

3 large cooking apples

12 dried apricots, finely chopped

4 thyme sprigs, leaves picked

1 tbsp butter or coconut oil, melted

For the crumble topping:

80g wholewheat flour

80g porridge oats

60g sunflower seeds

20g flaxseeds

50g cold butter, cubed

60g demerara sugar

Preheat the oven to 170°C Fan (190°C/375°F/Gas Mark 5).

To make the crumble topping, combine the flour, oats, seeds and flaxseeds in a large bowl. Add the butter and, using your fingertips, gently rub the butter into the mix until it forms small breadcrumbs. Stir in the sugar.

Grate the apples (skin on) into a bowl, stir in the apricots, thyme leaves and melted butter (or oil) and stir. Press the fruit mix into the base of an ovenproof crumble dish and top with the crumble mix. Bake in the oven for 30–35 minutes, until golden brown on top and bubbling.

Remove the crumble from the oven and leave it to rest for 10 minutes, then serve.

Tip:

If you don't like the thought of herbs in your crumble, feel free to leave them out, or if you love herbs try using rosemary or sage instead of the thyme, for an alternative twist.

PRALINE NICE-CREAM
with Dark Chocolate and Hazelnut Drizzle

SERVES 2

This ice cream is so easy to make and is great fun to decorate with kids – getting them involved with cooking from a young age is a good way to get them trying new foods too. It's dairy free and has far less sugar than shop-bought ice cream. Plus, who doesn't love praline?!

60g dark chocolate (minimum 70% cocoa solids)

30g roasted hazelnuts or almonds, roughly chopped

2 ripe bananas, peeled, cut into 2.5cm pieces, and frozen overnight

1 tbsp hazelnut or almond butter

2 heaped tbsp good-quality cacao or cocoa powder

Melt the chocolate gently in a heatproof bowl over a pan of simmering water (making sure the bottom of the bowl doesn't touch the water). Remove the bowl from the pan, add the nuts and stir gently.

Blitz the frozen bananas, nut butter, and cocoa powder in a blender or food processor until smooth.

Drizzle the chocolate over the ice cream, or stir through if preferred (it'll set quickly) and serve.

SPICED POACHED PLUMS

with Ginger Yoghurt and Toasted Almonds

SERVES 2

These warming flavours remind me of Christmas and fill the house with an incredible smell. You can use the same liquid to poach other fruits, such as pears, but you may need to adjust the cooking time slightly. The yoghurt is a source of calcium and protein and helps to cut through the sweetness of the plums.

For the plums:

4 ripe plums, halved and stones removed

200ml red wine

50ml water

½ cinnamon stick

1 clove

1 star anise

Pinch of ground ginger

To serve:

200g Greek or natural yoghurt

1cm piece of fresh root ginger, peeled and grated

Large handful of flaked almonds, toasted

Put the plums, wine, water and spices in a medium saucepan. Bring to the boil, then reduce the heat, pop on the lid, and simmer for 3–4 minutes, or until the plums are soft.

When the plums are almost completely soft, take off the lid, increase the heat and boil rapidly to reduce the liquid by half. Transfer the plums to a warmed bowl and strain the poaching liquid into a jug.

To serve, mix the yoghurt and ginger together, divide between two bowls, top with the warm plums and spoon over the poaching liquid. Finish with the toasted almonds.

Tip:

If you are vegan, coconut yoghurt works well with this, in place of Greek or natural yoghurt.

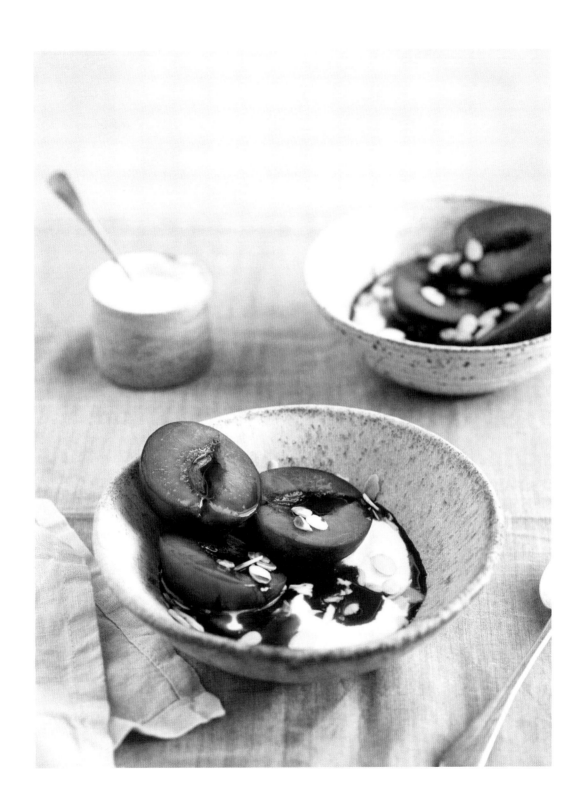

CACAO, MINT AND HAZELNUT POTS

SERVES 3–4

Mint and chocolate are delicious in these pots, and the creamy chocolate topping combines with a crunchy base to create perfect textures. It's easiest if you assemble the pudding in the pots, cups or ramekins they'll be eaten from, as it can be a little tricky to get the pudding out of a single tin in one piece. The pots can easily be altered to make them vegan (see tip).

For the base:

30g porridge oats

30g hazelnuts, chopped

30g buckwheat groats, soaked overnight and drained

20g honey

30g butter

For the topping:

3 tbsp good-quality cocoa powder

2 tbsp Greek yoghurt

1 ripe avocado

1 tbsp honey

5 mint sprigs, leaves picked

Preheat the oven to 180°C Fan (200°C/400°F/Gas Mark 6).

Mix the oats, hazelnuts and groats together then spread them out on a baking tray. Bake in the oven for 10–15 minutes, stirring them often so they don't burn.

Melt the honey and butter in a large saucepan, then add the baked oat mixture and mix well.

Divide the mixture between three or four pots, cups or ramekins (depending on how big your pots are), press it down very gently, and place the pots in the fridge to cool.

When the base mix is cold, put the ingredients for the topping in a blender and blitz until smooth. Spoon the mixture over the cooled bases and serve immediately.

Tip:

If you would like to make this vegan, simply swap the butter for coconut oil, the honey for maple syrup and the yoghurt for your favourite vegan yoghurt such as coconut or silken tofu.

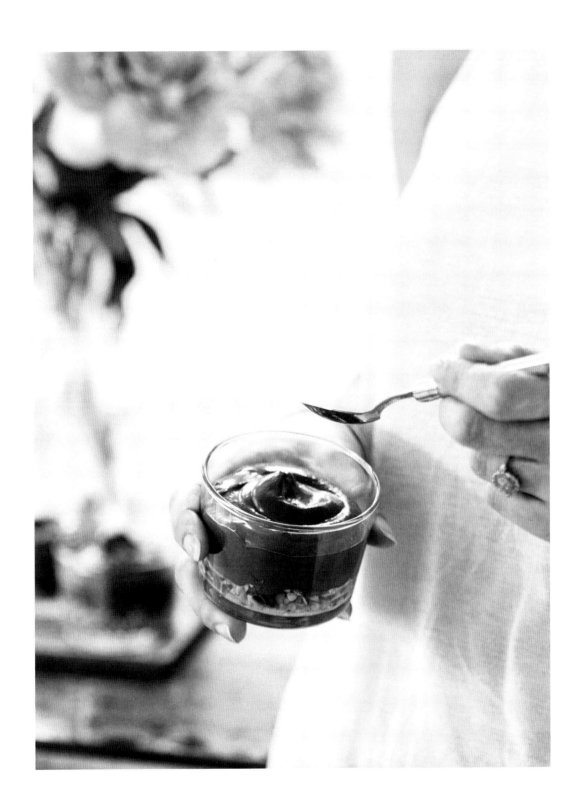

ROAST FIGS
with Orange, Honey and Pistachios

SERVES 2

Figs are sweet, fragrant and have the most beautiful flesh. When they are roasted they absolutely come alive, and orange further brings out the fruit's incredible flavour. The pistachios add texture to the dessert – it is a great dish for the end of the summer when figs are at their best.

4 ripe figs

2 tsp orange blossom honey (or similar)

½ tsp grated orange zest

2 tbsp yoghurt (optional)

2 tbsp pistachios, lightly crushed

Preheat the oven to 160°C Fan (180°C/350°F/Gas Mark 4).

Cut the nub off the top of each fig and cut a cross into the top of each to about halfway down. Using your fingers, squeeze the figs to force the cross to open up further so you can see inside the fig. Lay them, cross-side up, on a baking tray and drizzle the honey and scatter the zest inside each fig.

Bake in the oven for 10–12 minutes, or until soft, then serve in bowls with the yoghurt, if using, and pistachios scattered on top.

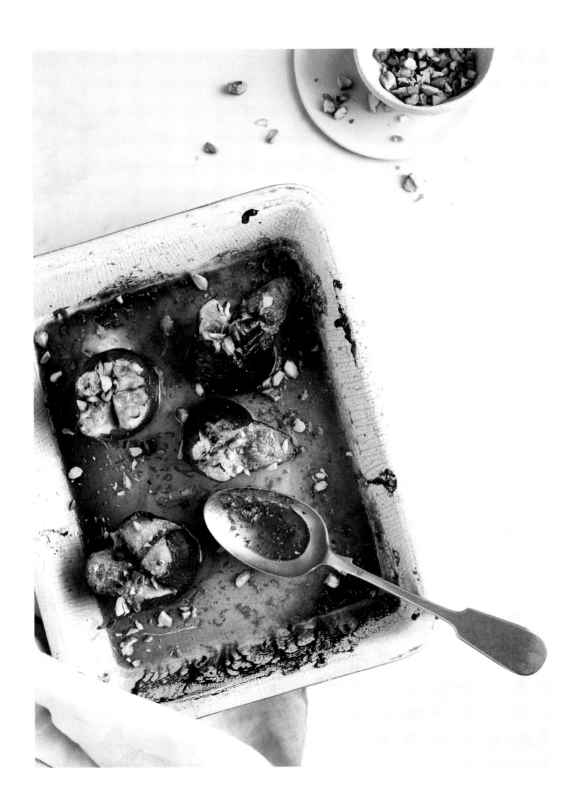

STRENGTHEN

STRENGTHEN

Welcome to your Strengthen chapter. This is all about getting your body strong, functional and flexible. I first discovered Pilates seven years ago and it was a real lightbulb moment for me. After spending years slogging away at the gym or pounding the pavements, which I didn't really enjoy, Pilates felt so much more controlled and enjoyable. Pilates has been the most strength-changing method I have used and it really is the kindest thing you can do to your body. This chapter is designed to make your body the most functional, comfortable, flexible and pain free it can be. It's about fixing postural issues, reducing muscle imbalances and building a core that supports and assists you. It's about being kind to your body and loving it enough to want to protect it.

WHAT IS PILATES?

Often confused with yoga, which is actually very different, Pilates is a method that focuses on strengthening the body as a whole, reducing muscular imbalances and promoting joint mobility through flexibility. It's one of the most powerful forms of exercise I have personally tried and it's thoughtful, structured and disciplined – very different from some of the more aggressive, one-size-fits-all methods out there. Pilates is often associated with those with injuries, the elderly or pregnant women, due to the fact that it can be adapted for people of all ages and abilities, but this does not mean it is easy! The beauty of Pilates is that it can be challenging for everyone, be it your first lesson or your thousandth. It requires concentration and control and teaches you so much about how your body moves and works.

In this book, we will really only be seeing the tip of the iceberg with Pilates, so please feel free to explore it more at your leisure. Once we become more aware of our bodies, we can really start to target our workouts to what they need, not just what the current trend is. Initially used by dancers and gymnasts around the world as a way of creating a strong, lean, flexible body, Pilates is now gaining popularity among the masses for its kind approach to strengthening and stretching. In The Model Method, Pilates makes up your strengthen element of the plan.

THE HISTORY OF PILATES

Pilates was created by Joseph Hubertus Pilates, about whom there are many stories, some potentially more accurate than others, which I will attempt to summarise. Joseph was born in 1883 in Germany. He was a sickly child, struggling with rickets, asthma and rheumatic fever, and was apparently taunted with the nickname 'Pontius Pilates'.

He began to take an interest in studying various exercise regimens as a young boy, determined to rid himself of his health problems. The present of an anatomy book from a doctor sparked his interest in the human body. Joseph was particularly fascinated by the classical Greek ideal of the human body and the connection between mind, body and spirit.

By the age of 14, with a physique that was approaching the anatomical ideal he found so interesting, Joseph's body was used as an example in anatomical charts. As he grew into adulthood and his strength improved further, he became a competent gymnast, avid skier and boxer. Around 1912, Joseph emigrated to England and became a circus performer, boxer and self-defence instructor to police schools and Scotland Yard. His personal experiences and training were forming the basis of Pilates, as Joseph was beginning to believe that our modern lifestyles, bad posture and inefficient breathing were the cause of our poor health.

As an 'enemy alien' during the First World War, Joseph was imprisoned by the British, but he took the opportunity to train and strengthen his fellow prisoners using the methods he had created over the years. This formed the start of his method – named 'Contrology' at the time – and Joseph boasted that his fellow prisoners would leave stronger than when they came in. For the prisoners who were injured or bed bound, Joseph created a variety of pulleys, using bed-springs attached to headboards, to create a resistance-based workout that could be practised without leaving the bed. This was a very basic version of his later invention – the Reformer Machine.

After the war, Joseph returned to Germany, where he began working closely with dance professionals, most notably Rudolf von Laban, who influenced much of the dance we see today. Joseph was soon asked by German officials to train the German army. Unhappy with the request, he decided to leave Germany for good.

In 1926, Joseph emigrated to America and with his new wife, Clara, set up a fitness studio, which happened to share an address with the New York City Ballet. This incredible location, and Joseph's growing reputation, created a busy studio, and his techniques began to spread further afield to dance classes across the US. Joseph Pilates, still in incredible shape, continued to teach clients at his studio right up until his death in 1967 at the age of 83.

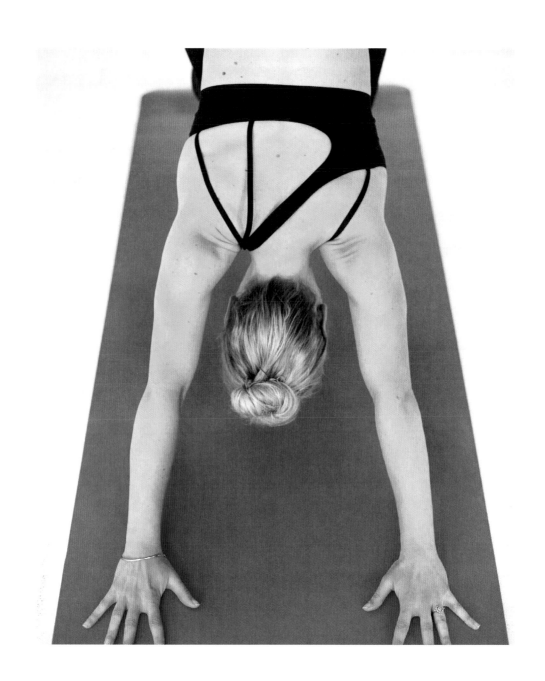

PILATES AND THE MODEL METHOD

In this book, I have listed some of my favourite dynamic Pilates exercises. I have taken some of the classical repertoire and tweaked it to give it a modern twist. This book is designed so that your workout can be personalised to you. You will need no equipment, other than a yoga mat, and will be practising your Pilates exercises every other day (three days per week) for 15 minutes, on the days you are not practising your HIIT.

I'll be giving you all the tools to discover how to read your body, decide what it needs and know how to adapt exercises to suit you. There is no one-size-fits-all approach to Pilates, and what I love most about The Model Method is that it is always tailored to your body and your body alone. I believe that to build lifelong wellness we need to really understand how the body works. So take time to read through the next few pages and learn all about your anatomy, muscle imbalances and postural type before choosing which exercises are right for you.

Glossary of terms in this chapter:	
Neutral pelvis	Your hip bones and pubic bone all lying on the same plane, whether lying or standing
Imprint	Your pelvis tilted backwards slightly bringing your hip bones and ribs closer together
Crucifix	Arms extended out to the side of your body as if you are a crucifix
Tabletop	Your legs should be lifted off the floor so that there is a 90 degree angle at your hips and knees. It is as if your shins are a table

ANATOMY 101

We are born with approximately 350 bones in our bodies. As we develop many of these bones fuse together, and by puberty our skeleton is made up of around 206 of these bones plus tendons, cartilage and ligaments. The skeleton is built to create an incredible mechanism for movement while being strong, versatile and having the ability to repair itself. The skeleton is not alone in these roles and works closely with the body's muscles, tendons and ligaments to facilitate a wide range of movement.

The role of the skeleton, however, is much more than simply movement. The skeleton is firstly vital for protection and support of our organs. The strength of the skeleton and the layout of our bones work to protect us whilst we engage in our daily movement as well as tough knocks and falls. The skull, for example, holds and protects our brain, providing a shock-absorbing and tough exterior for one of our most important and delicate organs. The ribcage protects our heart and lungs, and our vertebrae protect our spinal cord. Without the skeleton, not only would we be a floppy mess on the floor but our organs would risk daily damage from a mere trip or stumble. Our bones are also used for storage, and many of the body's vital minerals are held inside their central cavities. Calcium, phosphorus and many more minerals are released from the bones into the bloodstream as and when needed. Blood cells are also formed in the cavities of specific bones.

The function we will focus on most, however, is how the skeleton is moved. Pilates is focused around how our bodies move and how our skeletal system has adapted as a consequence of our lifestyle and health. I will discuss how, when you're working out which exercises will benefit you most; it's important to know how your muscles move your body.

JOINTS

Bones are connected to one another through a complex system of muscles, tendons, ligaments and cartilage. Tendons are strong, fibrous structures made of dense connective tissue that secure muscles to bone, facilitating bone movement. Ligaments are made of similar tissue but connect bone to bone, thus providing support to a joint. Cartilage has many different forms but is present in all of our joints. In some joints, such as our knees and wrists, it acts as a shock absorber between the bones.

Just as bones come in many different shapes and sizes, so do joints. Not all bones look like the archetypal long dog-toy-style bones we see in cartoons. For example, the bones of the spine, which are called vertebrae, look like an octopus from above and are irregular in shape. Some structures are formed by flat bones that have fused together, such as in the skull. Different bone shapes work together to give the skeleton structure but they are all fundamentally working to a similar purpose.

Almost all the bones in the body are connected to another bone via a joint. Each joint has a set range of movements it can do, and it cannot move comfortably outside that range (note that some joints allow no movement whatsoever). The type of joint at each connection dictates the movement allowed, and ligaments and tendons help to control and support such movement. Let's take the knee as an example. The joint at the knee is called a 'hinge joint'. It allows only flexion, extension and a very small degree of rotation, which enables the knee to lock out into full extension. If the knee is forced beyond its normal range of extension or rotation or into an abnormal movement such as side flexion (which is very common in sports such as rugby and tennis), the joint can be damaged. The movement it is forced into causes over-stretching, which can tear the fibres of the ligament or tendon. This then causes injury and prevents the ligaments and tendons from stabilising the knee.

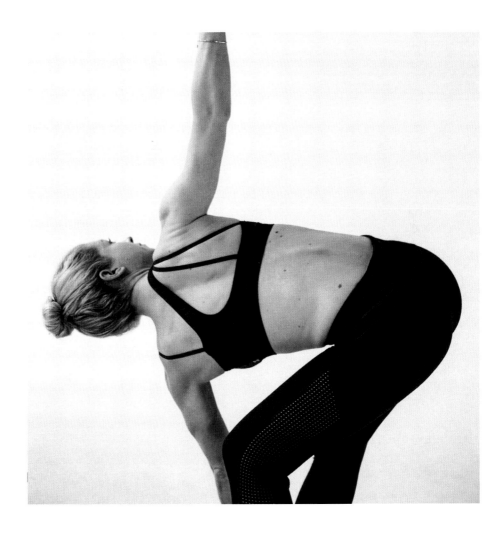

While joints allow certain movements to occur, it is our muscles that cause the movement. Muscles, making up around 40 per cent of our body weight, are formed of bundles of fibres that have the ability to contract (shorten) and relax (lengthen) in a coordinated manner, like elastic bands. Signals from the brain are passed down the spinal cord until they are able to pass their message on to a motor neuron that corresponds to the muscle requiring action. The motor neuron sends the message to the muscle fibres to contract and they do so, thus causing movement of the bones via the tendon (remember, tendons connect muscle to bone). The messages sent from the brain can either be voluntary (e.g. when we attempt to kick a ball) or involuntary (e.g. when the muscles in the digestive tract move food along the intestine). Involuntary muscles work with no conscious effort from us and are completely automatic.

We know that when we move our body a muscle has shortened. This muscle is called the 'agonist', and it caused the movement. However, there is always a muscle working against it – this is called the 'antagonist'. Imagine two people playing tug of war with a long rope. These two people represent two muscles that are both working against each other to keep a joint still. Let's say they are both as strong as each other and so the rope doesn't move at all. This is the equivalent to a joint staying perfectly still. Now, if one of those people gets stronger, the rope will move in their favour. The other person will have to be weaker and therefore have to allow the rope to move. So, for one person to 'win' and move the rope, the other person has to be weaker and allow the movement to occur. This is similar to what happens when a joint moves. One muscle will get a signal from the brain that tells it to shorten. The other muscle (which opposes it) will not get such a message (or will receive a weaker signal) and therefore the joint will move in favour of the stronger muscle.

An example of this is when we perform a bicep curl. Imagine your arm is straight down by your side with a dumb-bell in your hand. If you were to bend at the elbow to lift the dumb-bell closer to your shoulder, your bicep muscle would be shortening to do so, and therefore it would be your agonist. To allow the movement to occur, however, your tricep muscle has to lengthen – this is your antagonist. Most joints will have various muscles working to allow them to move; however, to keep it simple, try to imagine the agonist and the antagonist. If we use this explanation, we can understand why our bodies end up in uncomfortable positions if an agonist becomes too strong and an antagonist too weak.

It is important to know our muscles so we can understand which areas we need to work on. I often say to a new client, 'just engage your glutes a little', and frequently they'll ask me what their glutes are. This is completely understandable and I only know what they are because I work in fitness. There are hundreds of muscles in the human body and everyone will have a different opinion on which ones should be listed in this book. I have chosen to detail the ones I talk about the most in classes and the ones that can be described in a way that we can all relate to.

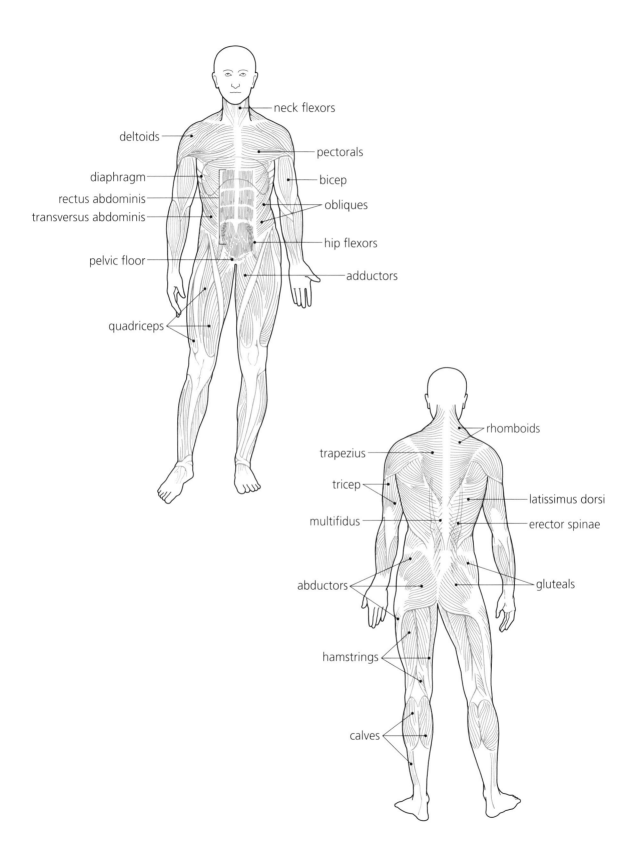

neck flexors

deltoids

pectorals

diaphragm

bicep

rectus abdominis

transversus abdominis

obliques

pelvic floor

hip flexors

adductors

quadriceps

rhomboids

trapezius

tricep

latissimus dorsi

multifidus

erector spinae

abductors

gluteals

hamstrings

calves

YOUR MUSCLE GUIDE

HAMSTRINGS *(semitendinosus, biceps femoris, semimembranosus).* The hamstrings are a collection of three muscles that run from the pelvis to just below the knee. They work to flex the knee (bend it) and to extend the hip (come out of a bend at the hip). An example of when we use the hamstrings is when we are cycling – the pulling of the foot upwards works our hamstring. Another example is when we play football and pull our leg back from the hip ready to kick a ball.

PELVIC FLOOR. These muscles act as a sling inside the pelvis, running from the pubic bone to the base of the spine and the two ischia (hip bones). They hold your pelvic organs in place and are involved in the process of passing urine. Weak pelvic floor muscles can cause incontinence and insensitivity during sex. We use them a lot in Pilates, in conjunction with contraction of the transversus abdominis to support the lower back and pelvis.

GLUTEALS *(gluteus maximus, gluteus minimus, gluteus medius).* This is effectively your bum. It's the round muscle at the top of your leg and at the base of your back that you sit on. Most people are unaware that the gluteal muscles (often called the 'glutes') are made up of three muscles. They, much like the deltoids do for the shoulder, provide movement at the hip, including extension, lateral rotation, medial rotation, adduction and abduction. They are also hip extensors, which means that they help to unfold the hips. They are used when we come from sitting to standing, like in a squat exercise. The hip flexors are the opposing muscles.

ABDUCTORS *(gluteals, tensor fascia latae).* These muscles, which include the gluteals, work to abduct the leg (which means they take the leg out to the side, away from the midline of the body). They run down the outside of the leg and spread themselves out from hip to knee. They can often be underused as we very rarely kick our leg out to the side whereas many of us naturally do the opposite a lot – crossing our legs.

ADDUCTORS *(adductor brevis, adductor longus, adductor magnus, adductor minimus, gracilis, pectineus).* The adductors run along the inside of your legs from near the pubic bone and down towards the knee so that as they shorten they bring the leg closer to the pubic bone. They are responsible for pulling the legs towards each other and can be felt when you squeeze a ball between your knees. They do individually have other actions on the leg or pelvis but we will not go into detail about those here. The abductors oppose these muscles.

HIP FLEXORS *(iliopsoas, psoas major, iliacus).* These muscles cannot be seen superficially as they are deep within the body, attached to the spine or pelvis and the femur (upper leg). These muscles are responsible for flexion at the hip. This means that, if I were standing and lifted up my left leg, my left hip flexors would be working. It also means that when I lie down and try to sit up (flexing at my hips), they are also working. Hip flexors can become short over time if we have a sedentary job; you can read more about this on page 131.

QUADRICEPS *(vastus medialis, vastus lateralis, vastus intermedius, rectus femoris).* These muscles take up the front of the thigh. Together they work to extend the knee (straighten the leg) during such exercises as squats, running and jumping. They collectively cover the area from hip to knee and can usually be felt when the leg presses against a weight.

CALVES *(gastrocnemius, soleus).* These muscles are located at the back of the lower leg and run from just below the knee and down to the achilles tendon by the heel. The gastrocnemius is the larger and most bulbous muscle, and can usually be seen just below the knee. The soleus is a flat muscle that lies underneath it. Together they work to create plantar flexion in the ankle (pointing it like a ballerina) so when we walk they help to propel us forwards. The gastrocnemius also assists in flexion of the knee joint.

ERECTOR SPINAE *(iliocostalis, longissimus, spinalis).* The erector spinae (split into three muscles) are incredibly important muscles for posture. They work together to extend the spine, which means that they are the muscles used when we move from a hunched-back position to a straight-back position. They work to maintain the neutral curvatures of the spine (see page 127) while we are standing and sitting, and without them our spines would collapse forwards under the pressure of gravity. They also work to laterally flex the spine, which means to bend it to the side (making you look like a crescent moon). In those with poor posture, this group of muscles is often weak and/or long.

OBLIQUES *(externus abdominis, internus abdominis).* Together, these muscles draw an X shape across the tummy. They work to compress the abdomen but most noticeably they rotate the trunk and/or bend the body to one side (lateral rotation). They work together to control movement of the trunk and pelvis and can be felt, and sometimes seen, as a line from the waist down towards the pelvis.

RECTUS ABDOMINIS. This is the muscle that we associate with six packs. The muscle looks like two elastic bands that run vertically from the pelvis up to the ribcage. Its role is to flex the lumbar spine (such as in a sit up, when we bring the ribs towards the hips) and to depress the ribcage (such as in forced expiration). It plays a vital role in stabilising the pelvis during walking and is an important postural muscle.

TRANSVERSUS ABDOMINIS. This muscle acts like a corset around your core and sits between the pelvis and ribcage. Because of its shape, it has the ability to compress the abdomen and provide support to the lumbar region. In Pilates, we try to engage it before certain exercises to attempt to maintain a neutral or 'imprinted' spine (see page 136).

MULTIFIDUS. These muscles are small but powerful. They attach from one vertebra to another like little support networks. They add stability to the vertebral joints, protecting them from movements created by the larger core muscles. They also aid extension (backwards bending), lateral flexion (side bending) and rotation of the spine.

BICEP *(biceps brachii).* The bicep can be felt at the front of your upper arm above the crease of your elbow. We can usually feel it move when we bend our arm, and it is often a visual muscle. It is used for flexing the arm and is worked harder the heavier the load in the hand is. An opposing muscle of the bicep is the tricep.

TRICEP *(triceps brachii).* The tricep can be felt, and often seen, running up the back of the upper arm, but it also has a connection across to the scapula (shoulder blade). This means that the tricep can help to adduct the arm bringing it into the body from crucifix (arms stretched out to the side like a crucifix) but it is most known for its ability to straighten the arm from flexed. It is used in the up phase of a push up as the arm is straightened.

LATISSIMUS DORSI. The 'lat' muscle takes up most of your mid to lower back. It runs from the spine and out to the front of the humerus (your upper arm). It works to adduct the arm (bring it from crucifix and back to your side), for example when you are trying to pull someone closer to you, and it also extends a flexed arm (straightens it).

PECTORALS *(pectoralis major, pectoralis minor).* The pectorals are effectively around where your breasts are. If you tense them, you may feel or see your breasts move. They work to draw the shoulder blades forwards (or apart from each other) and they rotate your arms forwards (medial rotation). When they are tight, we experience the classic 'hunched' look of shoulders that slump forwards and we lose the line of the collar bone. To reverse this symptom, we must work the opposing muscles (rhomboids and middle trapezius).

RHOMBOIDS *(rhomboideus major, rhomboideus minor).* These muscles run between the spine and the shoulder blades. They work to draw the shoulder blades together and also to stabilise them when the arms are moving. They are often long or weak in those whose shoulders have hunched forwards from working at a computer too much.

DELTOIDS *(deltoideus).* This is found at the top of the arm and can often be felt or seen as the bulb of muscles surrounding the shoulder socket. It is further broken down into three sections with differing roles – anterior (the front), middle and posterior (the back). These sections' jobs are to support the movement of the arm forwards, to the side and backwards. The shoulder has a huge range of movement and it is important that the muscles that support it are all strong to prevent shoulder pain or injury.

DIAPHRAGM. The diaphragm consists of muscle and fibrous tissue that separate the abdominal cavity from the thoracic cavity (containing the heart and lungs). It plays a crucial role in respiration as its contraction causes the thoracic cavity to expand, which draws air into the lungs. As the diaphragm relaxes, air is forced out of the lungs and expelled. In Pilates, the breath plays a large part in our exercises. You can read more about this on page 136.

TRAPEZIUS. The trapezius muscle is vast and takes up a large proportion of your upper back. It runs in a diamond shape from your neck down to your middle back and out to both shoulder blades. The upper fibres draw the shoulder girdle up towards the ears. These are often strong and/or tight in those with stressful jobs or who carry babies (they're heavy!) and can cause neck tension and headaches. The middle fibres draw the shoulder blades together, which is handy when so many of us are sat with them pulled apart during the day (e.g. when we work at a laptop). The lower fibres pull the shoulder blades down, especially against resistance. When we do pull ups (or hang from our arms), our lower trapezius works to stop the shoulder blades being pulled up too high and being damaged.

NECK FLEXORS *(scalenus anterior, scalenus medius, scalenus posterior).* These work together to flex your neck (the name gives it away, I guess) so they bring your chin towards your chest. You might feel these during tension in your neck when you do sit ups. Our heads weigh around 4.5 kilograms and when we practise sit ups the neck flexors have to work hard to prevent the head from falling backwards. This can be even more difficult for those who tend to hunch (kyphosis) as the back of their necks will be strong and the neck flexors will be weak.

MUSCLE IMBALANCES

Our bodies are designed in such a way that we can move, sit and walk safely and efficiently. In an ideal world, our bodies would maintain these ideal skeletal positions and we would all be healthy, happy, mobile individuals and back pain would be rare. Unfortunately, however, our lives have become more and more sedentary and the balanced musculature our bodies need for this 'ideal' body have changed and adapted over time. Our bodies initially evolved to allow us to stand tall, walk long distances and hunt and gather. With the increase in sedentary work and the rise of TV, social media and technology, we are spending increasing amounts of time sat down and less time walking. Most of us drive to work, sit at a computer all day, drive home and then sit and watch TV. We are no longer having to walk long distances each day and our bodies have started to adapt to this. What we are now seeing are people whose posture has completely changed due to their lifestyle.

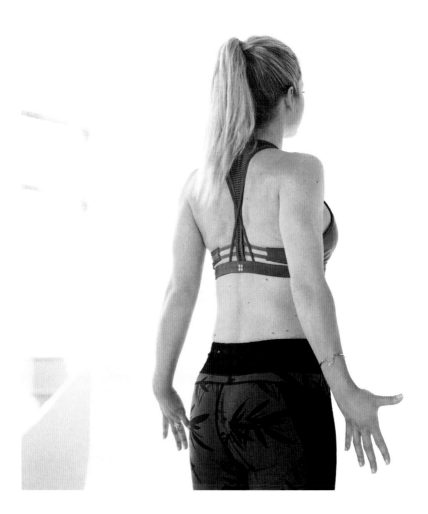

THE SPINE

Our spine is made up of 33 vertebrae, of which the top 24 are moveable, the vertebrae of the sacrum and coccyx are fused. The spine is further broken down into five regions based on their curvature (of which the coccyx and sacrum are two of the five). The illustration below shows the 'ideal' posture, which has three gentle curves of the spine that balance each other out. The head rests on the spine with the eyeline forwards.

- **The cervical spine.** With a weight of around 4.5 kilograms, the head is supported by the seven vertebrae of the cervical spine (your neck). It is incredibly mobile, which allows the vast range of movement we have at the neck. This part of the spine should have a gentle curve backwards (convex anteriorly) and our eyeline should be straight ahead.

- **The thoracic spine.** This is the largest part of our spine, with 12 vertebrae in total. The thoracic spine protects the heart and lungs and should have a gentle curve forwards (concave anteriorly). There is a limited amount of movement in the thoracic spine.

- **The lumbar spine.** This part of the spine bears the most amount of weight and it therefore has the largest vertebrae. The lumbar spine should have a gentle curve backwards (convex anteriorly).

- **The sacral and coccyx spine.** These are made up of vertebrae that have fused together. There should be no movement of these. They help to make up the pelvis.

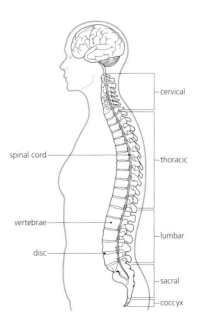

COMMON POSTURE TYPES

The illustration below shows some of the most common posture types. There are noticeable differences between each of them despite the fact that we are all made up of the same components and in theory have the potential to look like posture A (the 'ideal' posture type). Posture is a great indicator of your lifestyle, job and habits. You might find that you recognise one of the postures as being similar to yours straight away. You may, however, be totally unsure. Feel free to ask a friend or partner to help you assess whether you have any postural deviations (I know it's not exactly a sexy task to ask your partner, but they see you more than you see yourself). You could even take a photo. Sometimes you have to take a step back to see what your posture type is truly like. Another way to find out which postural type you are is to lie flat on the floor or stand flat against a wall. Feel which parts of your spine have the most contact with the floor or wall and then look at the chart to work out which type you are.

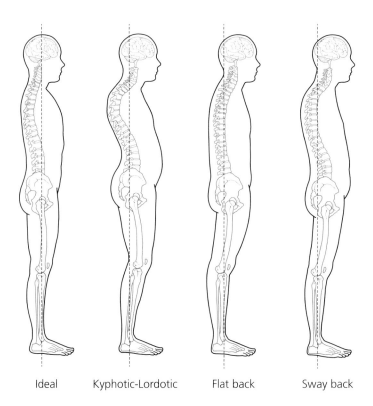

Ideal   Kyphotic-Lordotic   Flat back   Sway back

This is not an exhaustive set of postural deviations, but they are the most common. If you do fall into any of these types, read the following sections to learn what that means for your muscles to help you establish where you could focus your training first. The main reason for beginning here is so you know your limitations and can avoid injury while working up to have maximum movement and more importantly, controlled movement in all 24 joints of your spine, not just the areas that you naturally move more from. This will enable you to strengthen your body in a way that is safe and will help you avoid creating muscle imbalances.

KYPHOTIC–LORDOTIC

This is the posture type I see more than any other. Kyphosis and lordosis are two separate issues but it's common to see them both in the same person. Let's look at kyphosis first. If we look back at image B, we can see that, compared to our ideal posture, there is a very deep curve in the thoracic spine. We are supposed to only have a gentle curve and if it's exaggerated we end up with this hunchback-style posture. With the increase in curvature of the thoracic spine, we have to work harder to pull our heads back and so we can end up with a curve in the back of the neck that is also too great. If you are a computer user you may recognise this. It's common in those who slump at a desk looking at their computer or lean over for work (think masseuse or hairdresser). It's also common in people who are very tall who try to appear shorter or look down to speak to people a lot, and in women with large breasts. This type of posture makes it very difficult to stand up straight as the muscles in the back weaken and lengthen. The overextended neck can cause migraines and neck tension, and can be identified by a crease in the skin at the back of the neck.

- **Muscles to strengthen:** upper back extensors, erector spinae, neck flexors, middle and lower trapezius.

- **Muscles to stretch:** neck extensors, pectorals, rectus abdominis.

- **Exercises to practise:** Swimming (page 164), Kyphosis Corrector (page 166), Dumb Waiter (page 176).

If we now look at the lordosis element, we can see why people often have both kyphosis and lordosis. Kyphosis causes our thoracic spine to bend forwards more than it should. If we were to simply allow that to happen, we would be falling forwards often and lose our sense of balance. Our lumbar spine, in an attempt to help, tries to counterbalance this and deepens its curve too. If we look at the illustration opposite, we can see that the gentle curve in the lower back is also too deep and that the pelvis has tilted forwards. As this happens, it causes the lower back muscles to tighten and can be felt as lower back pain when standing for long periods of time. It is not always paired with kyphosis and often happens during pregnancy, where the weight of the baby pulls the spine into lordosis. It can also happen to those who have very tight hip flexors. I have quite extreme lordosis and it can be seen as me sticking out my bum and my tummy at the same time.

- **Muscles to strengthen:** external obliques, rectus abdominis, glutes.

- **Muscles to stretch:** hip flexors, lumbar extensors, hamstrings.

- **Exercises to practise:** Scooter (page 146), The Hundreds (page 154), Criss-cross (page 158).

FLAT BACK

When someone has a flat back, it means the natural curve in their lumbar spine has been reduced, effectively flattening it slightly. Having curves in our spine help with shock absorption, load bearing and balance. Flattening out these curves is not a positive thing. Unlike in lordosis, the pelvis has tilted backwards and flattened the lumbar spine. This is often associated with overactive abdominals (people who have spent years doing sit ups can experience this) and tight hamstrings. The hip flexors lengthen out and become weak and the thoracic spine may slightly change in reaction to the lumbar changes.

- **Muscles to strengthen:** lower back extensors, lower rectus abdominis, hip flexors.

- **Muscles to stretch:** hamstrings, abdominals, upper rectus abdominis.

- **Exercises to practise:** Single-leg Lifts (page 150), Scissors (page 160), Hip Twist (page 168).

SWAY BACK

In a sway-back posture the pelvis is tilted backwards yet it is also pushed forwards further than it should. Due to this tilt, the lower back flattens off and gives the appearance of leaning backwards. To prevent you from falling backwards, your thoracic spine bends further forwards (as in kyphosis) and your head juts forwards to compensate. It looks as if you are pushing your hips forwards, pushing your back backwards and then hunching over. The hip flexors and upper back extensors are stretched and the hamstrings are tight.

- **Muscles to strengthen:** hip flexors, upper back extensors, external obliques, middle trapezius.

- **Muscles to stretch:** hamstrings, pectorals.

- **Exercises to practise:** Single-leg Lifts (page 150), Criss-cross (page 158), Kyphosis Corrector (page 166), Cactus (page 172).

THE EFFECT OF A SEDENTARY LIFE

If I were to spend 12 hours of every day bicep curling, aside from being absolutely bored, I'd have very strong biceps. Those biceps would potentially be stronger than the rest of my body, to which I would have given little attention. As we know, when we work a muscle it gets stronger and better at producing the joint movement it was designed to perform. If we aren't also strengthening the opposing muscle (the antagonist), we end up with an imbalance of muscles at a joint. When we think back to our tug-of-war analogy, this would mean that person A has become much stronger than person B and the rope will keep moving in person A's direction. But what if person B needs to win? If we only strengthen one muscle, our body will favour moving in that direction. We end up changing our natural posture simply because person B is too weak to keep up. The same can also be said for muscles that are kept in a shortened position for too long. These muscles lose their elasticity and reduce our flexibility and range of movement at the joint, again changing our natural posture.

Let's see how these factors translate into some of the activities we do on a day-to-day basis.

SITTING AT A DESK OR ON A SOFA

When we are seated, we have flexion (a bend) at our hips, knees and ankles. The flexion in these areas means that the muscles that cross the joints are held in either a shortened or lengthened position. At the hips, our hip flexors are in a shortened position and our glutes are in a lengthened position. If we spend more time in this position than we do in the reverse position (which is standing up straight), our hip flexors will shorten over time and our glutes will get lazy and weak as they aren't being used.

At the knees, when we are seated, our hamstrings are in a shortened position and our quadriceps are in a lengthened position. Again, this can lead to tight/short hamstrings and weak/lazy quadriceps. Those who are sat down for much of the day become really good at sitting but really poor at standing. The muscles that help us stand up become weak and poor at their job and this is why many people feel lower back pain when they stand for too long.

Our mid to upper back (called our thoracic spine) is naturally concave anteriorly (i.e. the curve points backwards). This means that we are designed to have a gentle curve in our upper spine. This is to counteract the shapes of the lower back and neck, which curve the opposite way. If we spend too long leaning forwards looking over our phones or laptops, we start to pull the spine into an even deeper curve. Remember that gravity is also working against your upper back as it tries to pull you forwards, closer to the ground. The sheer weight of our upper body becomes increasingly difficult for our back muscles to support and so they become longer and weaker over time. Eventually the very muscles that help us stand up straight lose their ability to do so and we create a kyphotic spine (less affectionately known as a hunched back).

As a consequence of our backs starting to lean further forwards, we have to pull our heads back further to look up at our computer screens. This creates tension in the back of the neck, which can lead to headaches, migraines and shoulder pain.

TYPING ON A COMPUTER OR PHONE

When we are working with our arms in front of us, our shoulder blades separate to allow this to happen. The muscles that pull the shoulder blades together (rhomboids and trapezius) have to stretch to allow the shoulders to move forwards, and the arm rotates inwards in the shoulder socket to turn the palms to face down. Extended periods of sitting like this leave the shoulders hunched forwards (and often elevated up towards the ears), which is not only unflattering but also adds tension to the neck and shoulders.

BREASTFEEDING AND/OR CARRYING YOUR BABY ON ONE HIP

When we breastfeed or bottle-feed our baby, not only do we have to lean forwards and look down but we also have the weight of our baby in our arms, and babies are often quite heavy. This stretches the postural muscles of your upper back and can lead to tight muscles in the front of the body. The back of the neck lengthens as we look down at baby (much like looking down at your mobile phone all day) and weakens the muscles that lift the head back up.

If you carry your baby on one hip, chances are you are hiking up that same hip to prevent your baby from sliding off. This causes a tilt in your pelvis. The oblique (the muscles that draw the hips and ribs closer together) on the side doing the carrying have to work harder to support the weight of your baby but only on that side. Eventually you end up strengthening only one set of obliques and tightening or shortening the opposite set, along with one set of hip flexors and one set of muscles surrounding the spine. When you are no longer carrying your baby, you stand unevenly, mainly with your hips tilted to one side.

CARRYING A HEAVY HANDBAG

Women's handbags are thought to weigh around 2–3 kilograms on average. Imagine carrying that as a dumbbell all day – it would be obvious to presume that strength gains were going to be made. Carrying this weight in a handbag is the same! We tend to favour wearing our handbag on the same side every time and this forces us to work harder on that side to keep our shoulders level. This causes the obliques on the opposite side to work harder to pull the body back to that side (and to prevent you falling over to that side). As in the last example, once you take away the weight (the handbag), the imbalance in strength between your two sides can leave you with a spine or pelvis that tilts to one side.

SITTING CROSS-LEGGED

Women are often taught not to sit with their legs apart (hang in there – I know this is a weird sentence to start with). We attempt to look prim by crossing one leg over the other and it becomes a real habit that's hard to break. When you think about how awkward it actually is to sit that way, it's strange that we automatically do it so often. When we cross our legs, we cause our pelvis to tilt to one side. This tilt causes a shortening of the lower back muscles on one side too. We stretch the glutes and abductors on the leg that is brought across and squash the leg underneath. The adductors on your top leg are shortened and can tighten. Imagine what those effects look like when you try to stand back up normally again. A wonky pelvis will follow.

The above are just a few examples of common muscle imbalances in women. Although the potential changes they can cause might sound extreme, really in most of us they create only subtle changes. It is important to understand how your daily life affects your posture and start to make small changes to prevent your habits causing you discomfort. Remember that our skeletons were created to sit in a very specific way and pulling them out of their natural alignment, through injury or muscular imbalances, can cause aches and pain. At a more extreme level, these imbalances can pull the vertebrae into positions that cause slipped discs, trapped nerves and muscle atrophy (a wasting away of the muscle). Practising Pilates helps to ensure that underused muscles are not forgotten and tight muscles are given the freedom to stretch.

PREVENTING MUSCLE IMBALANCES

As we know, muscle imbalances occur when one muscle (or a group of muscles) is used more than another. Such imbalances cause movement in favour of the stronger muscle and the skeleton no longer sits as it should. The best way to prevent these imbalances, or at least reduce them, is to ensure you are working all the muscles of the body as equally as possible. Now, unfortunately we can't all just give up our desk jobs and enrol on an anatomy degree, but even just a little extra effort to strengthen otherwise weak muscles can make a huge difference! A big part of knowing which muscles to work is thinking about which movements you do on a day-to-day basis and reversing them. Take a moment to think really hard about what your day looks like for your body. What position do you find yourself in, and which muscles are being overused or shortened as a result? For example, if you sit hunched forwards all day, you'll be shortening the muscles in the front of your body and stretching your back muscles. You will most likely need to work the muscles that make you lean back (your back extensors). If you sit down all day in a chair, you'll probably need to work the muscles that make you stand up (your glutes). This does not mean, however, that you can't perform exercises that work the muscles in the 'tight' part of your body.

To make this topic even more confusing, just because a muscle is tight does not necessarily mean it is strong. One way to think of tight muscles that are weak is that they are shortened and cannot be used to their full potential. Back to the bicep curl example: if your biceps were tight and weak, you would only be able to perform a curl through mid-range as your muscle would struggle to move at its full range (or your body will try to protect the joint by limiting the movement). This would also mean the amount of power that can be generated is reduced.

When we work a muscle properly in Pilates, we are strengthening it but also making it more flexible. Therefore, if you have tight hip flexors, performing the Single-leg Stretch will strengthen the hip flexors but lengthen them too. Your best bet is to make sure you work as many muscles in the body as possible so they are all strong, functional and flexible.

The exercises in this chapter (see pages 140–181) are listed based on the area of the body they work. Each exercise lists the muscles that it targets and the benefits it has for your body. There is a description for each exercise that tells you who it is great for, but all the exercises in this book will benefit you in some way. You are the sum of all your parts and you want your whole body to be strong, so don't get too bogged down with worrying about which exercises are best for you if this all sounds confusing.

It's so important that we learn about how our bodies work, not only how they look! With all this information now in hand, spend some time getting to know your body – I mean really know it. Think about how it feels, what hurts, what feels great, what feels tight and what feels weak. Remember that our bodies change daily, so keep checking in with yourself.

A QUICK NOTE ON TECHNIQUE

Pilates is all about mindful, thoughtful movements. Try not to just rush through the exercises, speeding your way through them while thinking about work/dinner/the weekend. Really concentrate on what the exercise is for, why you are doing it, what muscles it's working and where you feel it. In Pilates if you are cheating, or using the wrong muscle, you are totally missing the benefits of the exercise. It is completely opposite to HIIT – I want you to move slowly and carefully. This may sound boring but it will make the exercises, and your muscles, work harder.

THE PILATES PRINCIPLES AND THE MODEL METHOD

Now that you have thought about what your posture type is, which parts of you are strong and which part of you are tight, you can start to think about designing your workout. I want you to spend 15 minutes a day, three days per week on your Pilates exercises. This might not seem much but exercise should not take over your life. Trying to fit in an hour every day would be so very hard to achieve and I doubt that routine would last very long. Pilates needs to be practised often but it doesn't need to take up your whole day. Aim for 15 minutes and if you happen to find you have a bit longer to spare, and most importantly you want to do a little more, then be my guest. Each exercise listed has the recommended number of repetitions next to it, so use this number as a guideline. Start with your warm up and then choose ten exercises you would like to do that day. If you run out of time, or end up with more time, adapt the number of exercises accordingly. Remember there are progressions and regressions to help you if you find the exercises too challenging or if you would like more of a challenge. Remember, technique is the most important thing here, so don't run before you can walk!

The Pilates Principles are the foundation of your Pilates practice. They are the focus points that should be considered before every exercise you complete. Thinking about each of these will become second nature and will ensure your technique is good and that you are feeling these exercises where you should.

THE BREATH

In Pilates there is a breath pattern for every movement. This can feel confusing at first but it is important and effective at allowing the correct muscles to engage. I have included the breath patterns with each exercise, but don't stress if at first you get them mixed up. Just keep checking in and it'll all become second nature in time.

In Pilates we breathe in through the nose and out through the mouth. When you inhale, try to take the breath into the sides and back of your ribcage so you really fill up your lungs. Most of us use a very shallow breath during the day, but in your workouts I want you to try to take the breath all the way to the lower lobes of your lungs. The abdomen will expand slightly on the inhale (however don't force this) and we will often inhale for the 'prepare' phase of an exercise rather than the movement.

When you exhale, you should feel your ribcage drawing in and down like a pair of bellows. You may feel that, as you do this, your spine tilts forwards slightly, and for this reason we tend to use the exhale for any spinal flexion (such as abdominal crunches). The exhale should be through pursed lips, almost like you are blowing out birthday candles, and so heard by others without causing tension in your face and neck. Visualise a light engagement of the core muscles throughout your breath.

PELVIC PLACEMENT

In most of the Pilates exercises I will mention your pelvic placement. There are two options with pelvic placement – 'neutral' and 'imprint' – and it's important for your back that you consider the placement of your pelvis before you move.

A neutral pelvis could be viewed as the ideal pelvic placement in that it is the position our pelvis should (or could) be if we had perfect bodies. It is how our pelvis was designed to be placed (however, very few of us have this placement), and in an ideal world we would want to be able to maintain a neutral pelvis throughout all daily movements.

To find your neutral pelvis, lie on your back with your knees bent. Take the heels of your hands and rest them on your hip bones. Take your fingers down to your pubic bone so you have drawn a triangle with your hands over your pelvis. Rock your pelvis backwards and forwards until your hands lie flat (imagine a cup of water in between your hands – would it spill or stay upright?). When those three points (hip bones and pubic bone) lie flat, you have your neutral pelvis. There should be a slight curve in the lower back without any feelings of tension. The tail bone should be heavy on the mat and you should feel relaxed.

To find your imprint, now tilt your pelvis towards you so that your pubic bone is a little higher than your hip bones. To do this, imagine a shortening of your obliques (so that your pelvis moves towards your ribs) and your lower back should lengthen slightly. Ensure that your tailbone is still heavy and has not lifted off the mat.

Take some time to find your neutral and imprint and start to memorise how each feels. You will need to be able to find your neutral when in other positions aside from lying, such as standing, lying on your side, and on all fours. It is the most stable and shock-absorbing position to be in and is often the main focus at the start of each exercise.

As much as we want to be able to work in neutral in most exercises, we tend to start in imprint if we are about to add a large load to our core, mainly when we are about to lie down with our legs in the air. It can be a struggle for many to maintain a neutral pelvis in this position so often your imprint pelvis will be safer and more stable.

RIBCAGE PLACEMENT

Our lower ribs are connected to our abdominals. The abdominals help to depress the ribcage and, therefore, if we ever find ourselves in a position where our ribcage has deviated forwards, or popped up, we can use our abdominals to bring them back to neutral. It is common for us to lose our correct ribcage placement during exercises involving movement of the arms or the thoracic spine, and even during normal breathing. Some movement of the ribs should be allowed, especially during inhalation or thoracic extension, but be wary of the ribs popping out uncontrollably or without care.

SCAPULA PLACEMENT

Our arms have a very large range of movement. They can reach forwards, sideways, overhead, behind us and even in circles. Compared to other joints of the body, their options are vast. The scapula (shoulder blades) act as an anchor for the arms and therefore are also involved in a wide range of movement. With the mobility we have at our shoulder, we must ensure there is stability of the scapula to match it. This is where scapula placement comes in. We must be mindful of where our scapulae lie before and during movements of our arms. Imagine width across the collarbone during movements and be mindful of the scapulae starting to creep their way upwards – as they do in so many of us in everyday life. The scapulae should lie flat on the back of the ribcage and smoothly glide across the ribs as you move, without poking out (winging).

HEAD PLACEMENT

Our cervical spine has its own curve, just like the thoracic spine and lumbar spine. We must ensure that we maintain this curve during movement. We should try to imagine the neck following the line of the spine so that it does not deviate from this neutral position. An example would be when we prepare for abdominal exercised such as an abdominal curl/crunch. Many of us may recognise this as being like a crunch. When we lift the head and shoulders, we should focus on the effort coming from the tummy, and the chin should not be jammed into the chest – the neck follows the line of the spine. Or, in the Kyphosis Corrector, when we lift our head and shoulders up away from the floor, we must make sure we do not fling our head back. In both of these examples, we will prevent neck tension by following these principles.

One way to ensure we keep tension away is to lengthen the back of the neck when we are about to lift it away from the mat (when lying on our back). We call this a 'head nod'. We are not digging the chin into the chest; we are simply lengthening the back of the neck enough to create a mini double chin. This will help you to maintain alignment. Try it in your Hundreds exercise (page 154).

So now you know the main postural principles, remember to consider them during each exercise. We want to make sure that we are working the correct muscles and not causing unwanted tension. Please also remember that there is a mind–body connection in Pilates. It is not mindless, so during your exercises think about where you are meant to feel the exercise, where you are actually feeling it and what the breath pattern is. No thinking about tomorrow's deadline or tonight's dinner – just the job in hand.

YOUR STRENGTHEN EXERCISES

Practise your Pilates exercises every other day (three days per week) for 15 minutes, on the days you are not practising your HIIT. Choose your Strengthen exercises based on your posture type, muscle imbalances or what you feel your body needs.

LOWER BODY DOMINANT

Arabesque Deadlift

Ship

Elevated Clams

Scooter

Side-lying Leg Raise

Single-leg Lifts

Single-leg Squat

CORE DOMINANT

The Hundreds

Single-Leg Stretch

Criss Cross

Scissors

Mermaid Plank

Swimming

Kyphosis Corrector

Hip Twist

UPPER BODY DOMINANT

Single-arm Push-up

Cactus

Leg Pull Prep

Dumb Waiter

Incline Push-up

Pilates Push-up

Throughout these exercises, 'regressions' are ways to make an exercise easier and 'progressions' are ways to make it harder.

ARABESQUE DEADLIFT

The arabesque deadlift is fantastic at lengthening and strengthening the posterior chain of muscles while challenging your balance and stability. The back muscles work isometrically throughout to maintain a neutral spine against gravity. Take care that you are slow and steady with this exercise as it is very wobbly. Visualise your return back to the start as you open up the front of the hips.

TARGET MUSCLES:

Hamstrings | Glutes *(to return the hips to start position)* | Spine Extensors | Quads | Core *(for stability)*

REPS:

8 on each leg

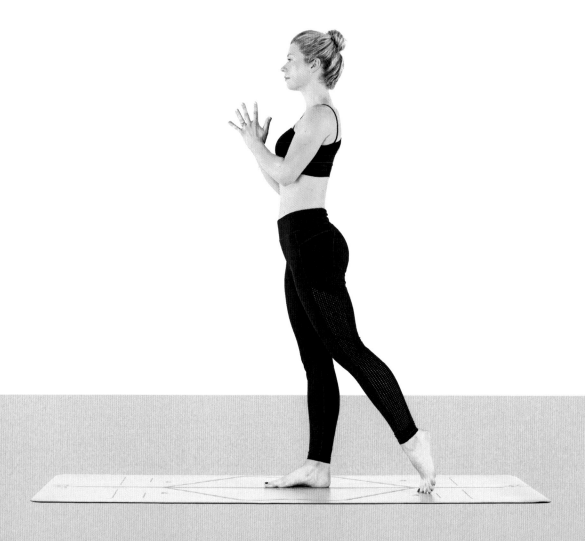

TECHNIQUE:

Stand with your weight on your right leg, ensuring your knee is soft. Take your hands to prayer at your chest or extend them out to crucifix. Ensure you have a neutral spine. As you inhale, begin to hinge the upper body forwards at the hips while lifting the left leg out behind you. You are aiming to bring your torso forwards to a 90-degree angle with your right leg while elevating your back leg up behind you to 90 degrees so that you resemble the letter T. Keep the movement slow and fluid. As you exhale, slowly begin to lift your torso and lower your left leg, until you come back to your start position. Repeat.

TEACHING POINTS:

Keep a soft bend in the supporting knee. Extend the back leg long. Keep the hips level. Keep the spine neutral.

REGRESSIONS:

If your balance is poor, try holding the back of a chair, a TRX, a ballet barre or table for support. You can also reduce the range of movement so you are only hinging at the hips by 45 degrees.

PROGRESSIONS:

Add a weight into the opposite hand (e.g. if you are weight-bearing on your left leg, put a weight in your right hand). You can also add a hold at the end while abducting your leg out to the side. Another possibility is to reach forwards and touch the floor for the last hold and lift the leg as high as possible using the glutes.

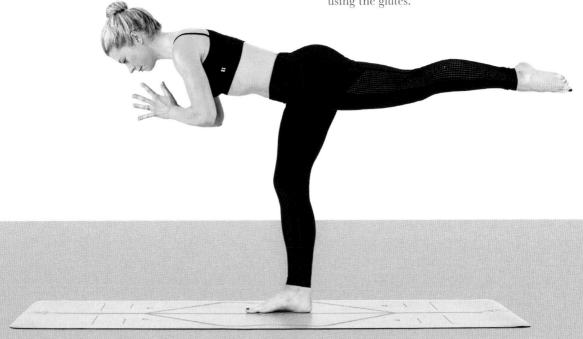

SHIP

This exercise is a great way of learning how to engage and relax the glute muscles while stimulating the deep muscles of the pelvis. The hip extensors hold the hips high while the obliques work to create a level pelvis. It's also a great way of opening up the front of the hips and stretching the hip flexors. Go slow and steady on this one and imagine you have a glass of champagne on each knee that you don't want to spill (of course).

TARGET MUSCLES:

Glutes *(to lift the hips)* | Obliques | Pelvic Floor | Hamstrings |
Hip Adductors | Hip Flexors | Spine Extensors

REPS:

10 on each side

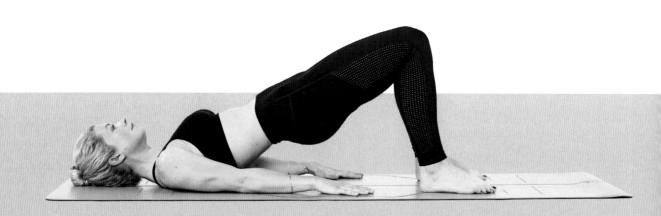

TECHNIQUE:

Start by lying on your back, knees bent comfortably with feet and knees hip-distance apart, and arms long by your sides. Inhale and as you exhale start to engage your glutes and roll through your spine one vertebra at a time to lift the hips up towards the ceiling. Stop when you feel that you are a diagonal line from shoulders to hips to knee. Ensure your knees are still hip-distance apart and your abdominals are engaged with no ribs poking out. On your next inhale, slowly release your left glute and let your left hip lower an inch. Exhale to carefully lift it back up in line with your right hip. Inhale and lower your right hip an inch. Exhale to lift it back up. Keep alternating from one hip to the other ensuring that the hip left behind stays perfectly still. Imagine the hips are a ship that is swaying from side to side at sea. Once you have finished your reps, inhale to hold and exhale to slowly, one vertebra at a time, roll your spine back down until you have returned to your start position.

TEACHING POINTS:

Ensure that your lumbar spine is in neutral (you should not have a deep arch in your lower back). The tummy should not be poking out and neither should your ribs. Keep the knees perfectly still and make sure the movement has come from the pelvis. Your weight should be on your shoulders, not your head or neck.

REGRESSIONS:

Practise the slow, methodical lifting of the pelvis first. Ensure you are able to lift the hips up one vertebra at a time until you reach your diagonal line. If you feel cramp in your hamstrings, it is usually a sign your glutes are slow to activate and/or you have tight hamstrings. Building up slowly will help.

PROGRESSIONS:

Once you are in your glute bridge, lift your left leg into tabletop. Keep it there as you lift and lower just your left hip. Once you have completed ten reps, swap the legs over and repeat with your right hip.

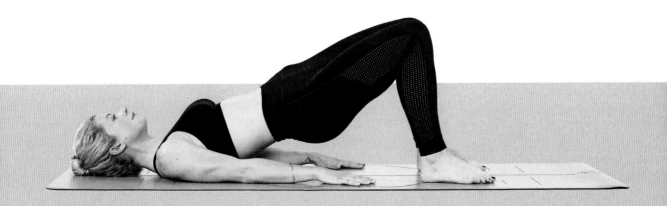

ELEVATED CLAM

The clam is great for those with lower back pain or hip injuries. It works muscles that are often neglected in everyday activities. How often do we stand with our knee bent and rotate our leg in the hip socket?! Rarely. So it's important to ensure that the hip rotators don't get ignored, especially as they play a key role in knee joint alignment. Strengthening the hips helps to support the pelvis when standing and this in turn supports the spine.

TARGET MUSCLES:

Gluteus Medius | Hip Abductors | Obliques *(to prevent rotation of hips)* | Core *(to lift the waist)* | Pelvic Stabilisers *(to keep the pelvis still)*

REPS:

10–12 on each side

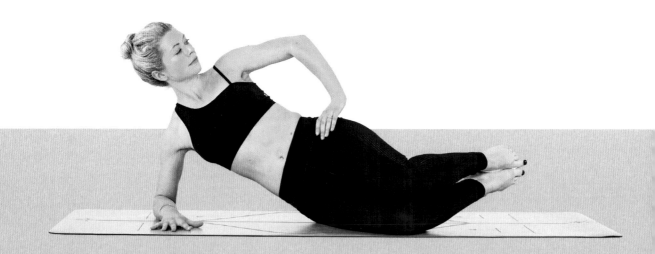

TECHNIQUE:

Lie on your right-hand side with your hips stacked one on top of the other, propping yourself up on your right forearm. You need to ensure you are not sinking into your right shoulder and try to keep a triangle of space between your ribs and the floor. Your knees and hips are bent and resting on the ground for support while your feet are lifted and connected. Inhale and as you exhale keep your feet together and rotate your left knee up towards the ceiling (externally rotating the leg). On the inhale release it back to the start and repeat.

TEACHING POINTS:

Ensure that your feet are not lifting further away from the floor – we only want rotation at the hip, not further elevation. Make sure that your pelvis stays still during the movement – don't rock back and forth with the movement. Watch that the shoulder does not creep too far to the ear as this will cause tension in the neck.

REGRESSIONS:

If it is a struggle to keep the leg lifted, lower the leg down after every 2 reps and build up until you are able to do 10–12 reps on each side.

PROGRESSIONS:

Try tying a resistance band around your knees before you separate them. This will create resistance on your top leg and you will have to work harder to lift the top knee. This will engage the hip abductors more.

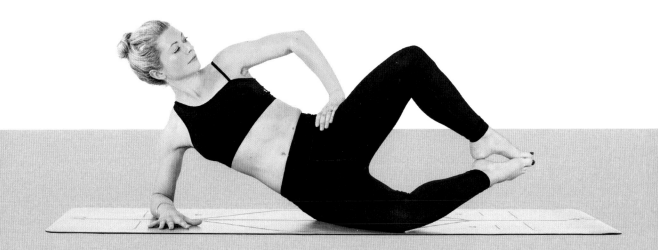

SCOOTER

This exercise is fantastic at engaging the glutes, especially in those who struggle to 'feel' them or end up feeling fatigue in their quadriceps before their glutes have had a chance to warm up. The key here is to keep the weight in the heel of the standing leg as much as possible and sit so far back you fear you may fall backwards – almost as if you were sat on a scooter or moped. If the weight creeps into the toes, you will feel this in your quads. Keep the hips level and go slow.

TARGET MUSCLES:
Quadriceps *(to stabilise knee)* | Glutes *(to maintain squat position)* | Back Extensors | Hip Stabilisers *(adductors and abductors)* | Obliques and Multifidus *(to prevent rotation)* | Core Muscles *(to maintain neutral alignment)*

REPS:
8–10 on each leg

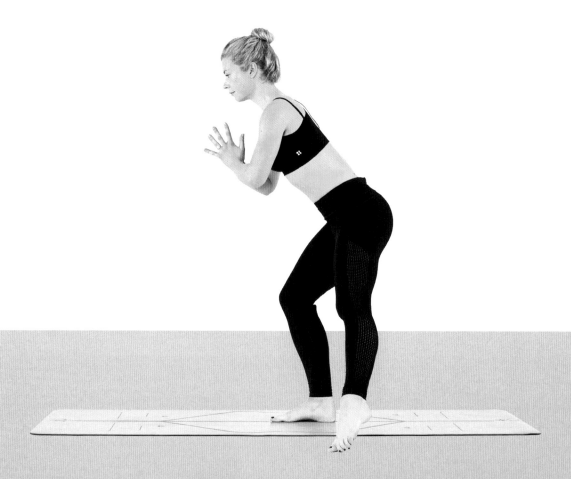

TECHNIQUE:

Start by sitting down into a mini squat, ensuring your weight is in the back of your feet. Make sure you have a neutral spine as you lean forwards slightly and take your hands into prayer at your chest. Take your weight over onto your right leg. Lift your left foot off the floor. Inhale and as you exhale stretch the left leg out behind you and tap the floor with it. Inhale to bring the leg back towards the start position and on your next exhale stretch it out to the side and tap the floor with it. This is one rep. Repeat until all reps are performed and then swap legs.

TEACHING POINTS:

Ensure you are engaging your core and pelvic floor to maintain a neutral spine. Try not to hunch or allow the shoulders to stoop forwards. Keep the toes of the supporting foot light and sit back. Ensure your supporting knee stays neutral and doesn't collapse inwards.

REGRESSIONS:

If you are finding this difficult, reduce the depth of your squat or to learn the choreography start in a standing position instead.

PROGRESSIONS:

Sit lower and at the end of your last rep take the leg out behind you and lift it off the floor. While doing so, lean your body closer to the floor while lifting the back leg as high as possible and hold for 5–10 seconds.

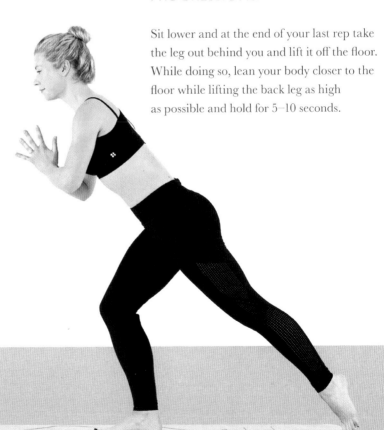

SIDE-LYING LEG RAISE

This is really effective at engaging the hip abductors, which play an important role in pelvic stability and knee alignment. If you are a runner, these are important for you and help to prevent the dreaded 'runner's knee'. If you notice that when you squat your knees collapse in towards each other, this exercise will be your best friend. Make sure you keep your pelvis still and only lift the leg as high as a neutral spine can be maintained.

TARGET MUSCLES:
Glutes | Hip Abductors *(to lift the leg)* | Core Stabilisers *(to maintain a neutral spine)* | Obliques *(to prevent rotation of the pelvis)*

REPS:
10–12 on each leg

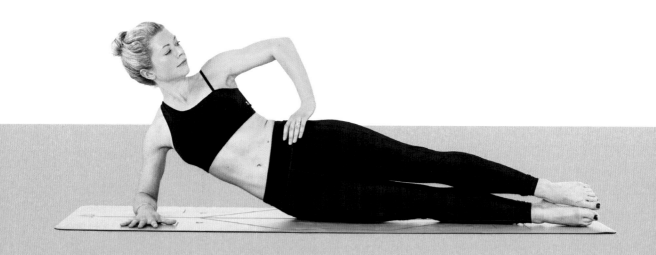

TECHNIQUE:

Start by lying on your right-hand side. You can rest on your arm as in the photo or if it's more comfortable take your right arm overhead (resting on the floor) and parallel to the rest of your body (like you are an arrow). Stack your hips on top of each other with nice straight legs. Ensure that your spine is neutral and that you are keeping a little gap between your waist and the floor – not simply sinking into the floor. Inhale and as you exhale lift your left leg slowly up towards the ceiling, as high as a neutral pelvis can be maintained. As you inhale, slowly lower the left leg as if there is imaginary resistance underneath it. Repeat.

TEACHING POINTS:

Imagine there is a beach ball between your legs as you lower your top leg back down. Keep the hips stacked and do not hitch your hips to the side as you lift your leg. The slower you move, the harder you'll work. Try to relax the upper body as much as possible.

REGRESSIONS:

Start with your legs slightly in front of your body, like a banana, to help you stabilise your hips better.

PROGRESSIONS:

Add an ankle weight or tie a resistance band or loop around your ankles to increase the resistance. If you are very advanced, you could attempt to lift both legs at the same time, but make sure you keep control of your pelvis and do not create tension in your neck.

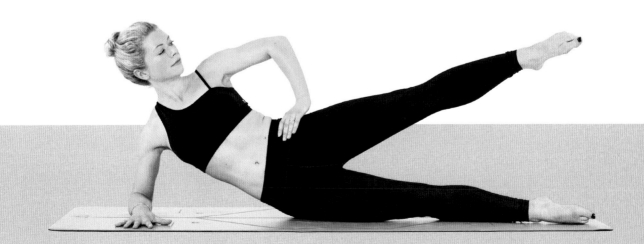

SINGLE-LEG LIFT

Tight hip flexors are incredibly common given that so many of us have sedentary lives. The more we sit down, the tighter our hip flexors become as they adapt to the shortened position. When we have tight hip flexors, we struggle to stand with a neutral pelvis due to the downward pull the hip flexors create. This exercise works on lengthening and strengthening the hip flexors while reducing the pull they have on the pelvis. We are aiming for long, strong muscles here, so technique is important on this one.

TARGET MUSCLES:

Hamstrings | Glutes | Hip Flexors *(to lift and lower the leg)* | Obliques *(to maintain a neutral pelvis)* | Transversus Abdominis *(to support the lumbo-pelvic region)*

REPS:

4–6 on each leg

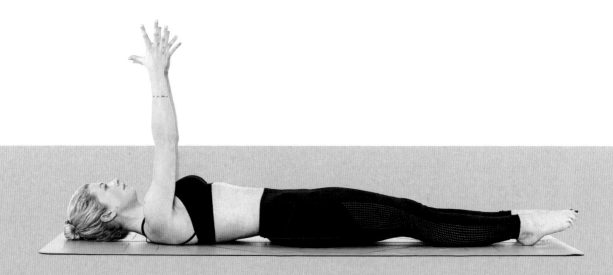

TECHNIQUE:

Lie on your back with your legs long, your head relaxed (on a pillow if more comfortable) and your eyeline straight up. Bring your hands to your pelvis and, using the technique described on page 136, find and maintain a neutral pelvis throughout. Bring your arms straight up to reach the ceiling. Inhale and as you exhale slowly lift your right leg away from the floor and up to the ceiling only as high as you can keep your leg straight. Remember you must keep a neutral pelvis. As you inhale, slowly lower the leg back to the floor. Complete all your reps on the left leg before switching to the right.

TEACHING POINTS:

The most important thing is that you keep a neutral pelvis throughout. If you struggle to get your feet off the floor without losing your neutral, try the regression until you are strong enough to move on to the standard version. Ensure you keep your leg straight as it lifts so you get a lengthening of the posterior chain too. Try to keep the tension out of the neck and shoulders and keep the effort in the core.

REGRESSIONS:

If you are struggling to maintain a neutral pelvis, aim for imprint instead – this will provide more support for the lower back. You can also start with your knees bent and lift the leg in its bent position. This will reduce the 'weight' of the leg and make it easier to maintain an imprint position. Some people find the initial lifting of the leg the hardest part so you can try starting with your left leg straight up in the air and lower it only as far as you can maintain neutral.

PROGRESSIONS:

When you lower the leg back towards the floor, stop one inch away from it – in other words, don't allow your leg to rest back on the floor between reps. The slower you move, the harder you work. If you are very advanced, you could attempt this with both legs at the same time but only if you can maintain control through your core and shoulders.

SINGLE-LEG SQUAT

The single-leg squat is great at challenging pelvic stability and strengthening the gluteus medius. The main challenge is maintaining a level pelvis and not allowing the hip to dip. The exercise is incredibly functional as it mimics everyday movements and can also highlight any strength differences between the legs (which are quite common). Be aware of what your knee does as it bends – try to keep it facing forwards and not collapsing inwards.

TARGET MUSCLES:

Glutes *(to lift the hips and maintain a neutral spine)* | Hamstrings | Quadriceps | Hip Flexors *(of elevated legs)* | Obliques

REPS:

8–10 reps on each leg

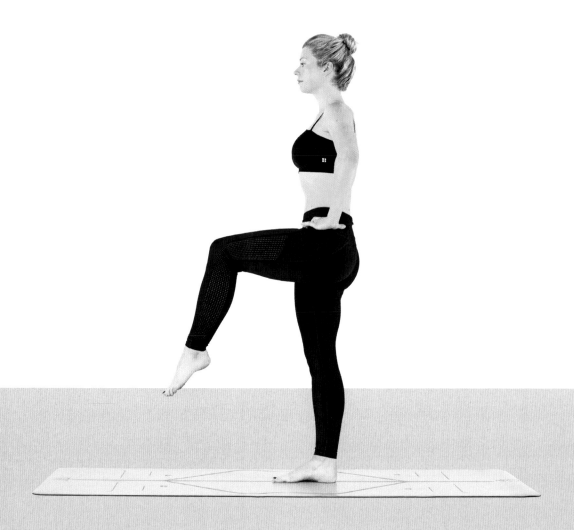

TECHNIQUE:

Stand in front of a chair, bed or stool (something you can sit down onto). Engage your core, transfer your weight to the right leg and lift your left leg up to a tabletop position. With hands on your hip bones to check they are level, inhale and start to bend your right knee, lowering your bum down with control onto the chair. As you exhale, press into the heel of your right foot and press yourself back up to standing. Repeat all your reps on this leg before switching to the other leg.

TEACHING POINTS:

Aim to keep the hips as level as possible while moving. Using a mirror will really help, or closing your eyes and 'feeling' the movement can be beneficial. Engage your core and move as slowly as possible to maintain control. Make sure you are not hunching over and keep the weight in the back of the foot.

REGRESSIONS:

Don't worry if you can't sit all the way down onto a chair, or can't get back up if you do. Simply reduce your range of movement and sit only half-way down until your strength builds up. If you struggle to maintain balance, keep the toe of your elevated leg gently on the floor for more stability.

PROGRESSIONS:

Get rid of the chair. This will give you a greater potential range of movement but be careful that you don't lose your technique.

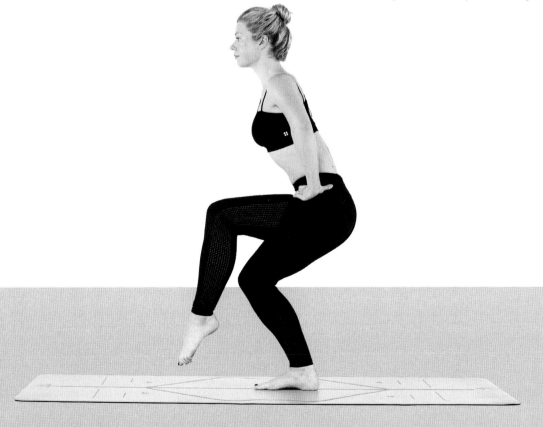

THE HUNDREDS

The Hundreds is a great exercise for building endurance of the abdominals. It is important to have strength in a muscle to create movement but it is muscle endurance that assists our bodies in maintaining ideal posture during the day. If a muscle has poor endurance, we can get into an ideal posture but struggle to maintain it for a prolonged period – think of how much we require our core strength during the day. Do not feel pressure to complete a whole hundred reps here – build up and maintain your technique.

TARGET MUSCLES:
Transversus Abdominis *(to support the lumbar spine)* | Pelvic Floor *(to assist the Transversus Abdominis)* | Rectus Abdominis and Obliques *(to create flexion of the upper back and maintain imprint)* | Scapula Stabilisers *(during movement of the arms)* | Adductors and Quadriceps *(for the progression version)* | Hip Flexors *(for the progression version)*

REPS:
50–100 pulses
(in one round)

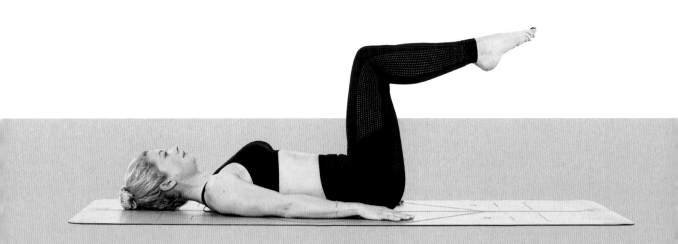

TECHNIQUE:

Start by lying on your back with your knees
bent and feet on the floor. Your arms should
be long by your sides and palms facing down.
Imprint your spine and take your left leg
into tabletop followed by your right. Inhale
to lengthen the back of the neck slightly
and as you exhale contract the abdominals
to flex your upper back and lift your head
and shoulders away from the mat. Your
arms should be lifted off the mat in line
with your shoulders, reaching towards the
feet end of the mat. On your next inhale,
maintaining the spine in flexion, make
small pulsing actions with your arms for five
counts. Exhale, pulsing for another 5 counts.
Continue with this breath pattern for the
remainder of your pulses. After 100 pulses,
inhale to hold, reaching further with the
arms, exhale to lower your head and rest.

TEACHING POINTS:

Make sure that you maintain imprint
throughout and try to keep the face and
neck as relaxed as possible to prevent too
much neck tension. Visualise the ribcage
drawing down towards the hip bones and
keep the collarbone wide. The arms should
be moved with intent but shouldn't cause the
body to bounce.

REGRESSIONS:

Keep the feet on the floor as in your start
position to reduce the pressure on the core
and hip flexors. If you find you get a lot of
neck tension during this exercise, take one
hand behind the head for support for half of
your pulses and then swap to the other hand.

PROGRESSIONS:

As you lift the head and shoulders to come
into your start position, also extend the legs
to a diagonal line. This will increase the
'load' for the core and challenge the hip
flexors. The lower the legs, the harder this
will be, but be careful not to lose imprint.

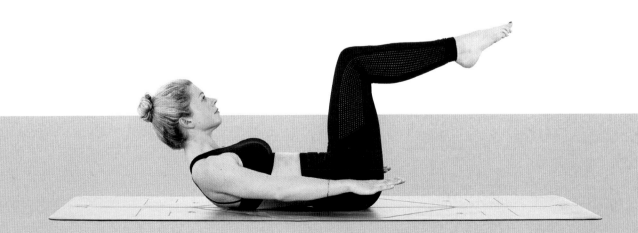

SINGLE-LEG STRETCH

The single-leg stretch is great for building abdominal strength and endurance while also challenging coordination and encouraging a lengthening of the hip flexors. It's also a great exercise to practise coordinating the breath with the movement, as each time you extend your leg you exhale. I really enjoy teaching this exercise and it's a fun exercise to do (in my opinion).

TARGET MUSCLES:

Transversus Abdominis *(to support the lumbar spine)* |
Pelvic Floor | Rectus Abdominis and Obliques *(to create flexion of the thoracic spine)* | Obliques and Multifidus *(to prevent excessive movement of the pelvis)* | Hip Flexors

REPS:

8–10

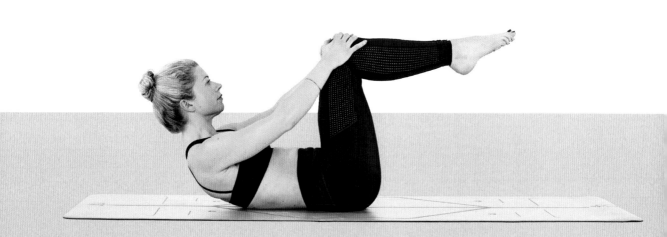

TECHNIQUE:

Start by lying on your back with your knees bent and feet on the floor, arms long by your sides. Imprint your spine and take your left leg into tabletop followed by your right. Inhale to lengthen the back of the neck and as you exhale contract the abdominals to flex your upper back and lift your head and shoulders away from the mat, bringing your hands to outside your knees. Inhale and as you exhale straighten your left leg out to the diagonal and bring both hands to your right knee. On the inhale begin to switch the legs and as you exhale straighten your right leg, bringing both hands to your left knee. Keep switching until you have completed your reps. Inhale to bring both legs in, exhale to relax your head and shoulders back down.

TEACHING POINTS:

Visualise the abdominals lying flat and ensure that you maintain imprint (unless attempting the progression). Try to prevent the pelvis rocking from side to side. Only allow the straight leg to go as low as you can maintain imprint (or neutral) and try to keep the tension out of the neck and shoulders. Don't let reaching for your knee cause you to hunch – keep the collarbone wide.

REGRESSIONS:

If you are struggling with the choreography for this exercise, attempt it with your head staying down on the floor and practising the leg and breath movements slowly. If it is a struggle to maintain flexion of the upper back without causing tension in your neck, reduce the number of reps until you feel only aching in your tummy and not your neck. You can then build up your reps.

PROGRESSIONS:

If you are strong enough, maintain a neutral pelvis throughout instead of imprint. Once you have perfected your breath-to-movement pattern, add in the arm choreography. As you straighten your left leg, bring your right hand to your right ankle and your left hand to your right knee. When you straighten your right leg, bring your left hand to your left ankle and your right hand to your left knee.

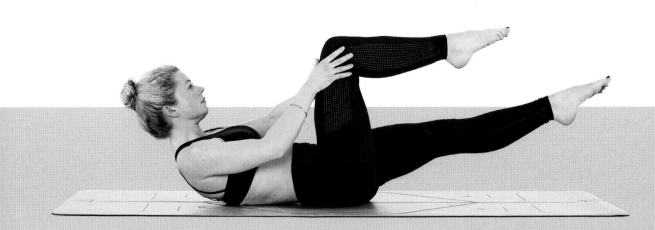

CRISS CROSS

This exercise is fantastic for targeting the obliques and adding some spinal rotation into your workout. This is an exercise I see people practising outside Pilates workouts and it's often very aggressive and ballistic. It should be a smooth, controlled movement with no bouncing or head banging. Obliques are great for stabilising the spine and pelvis, and assisting you when rotating or bending your spine to the side.

TARGET MUSCLES:

Obliques *(both external and internal, to create rotation of the spine)* | Transversus Abdominis *(to support the lumbar spine)* | Pelvic Floor | Rectus Abdominis and Obliques *(to create thoracic flexion)* | Hip Flexors

REPS:

8–10

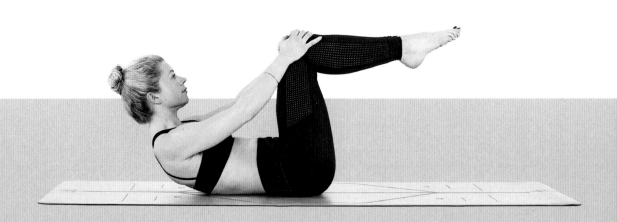

TECHNIQUE:

Start by lying on your back with your knees bent and feet on the floor and your hands resting behind your head. Imprint your spine and take your left leg into tabletop followed by your right. Inhale to lengthen the back of the neck and as you exhale contract the abdominals to flex your upper back and lift your head and shoulders away from the mat, keeping elbows wide and hands gently supporting the head. Inhale and as you exhale straighten your left leg out to the diagonal while rotating your upper body towards your right knee. Inhale to come back through the centre and as you exhale take your right leg out and rotate towards your left knee. After you have completed your reps inhale to hold and exhale to lower your head back down.

TEACHING POINTS:

Keep the elbows wide – you should only just be able to see them in the corner of your eye, with the collarbone wide and the neck and shoulders relaxed. Remember that we are rotating our spine not side bending, so no bouncing up to get your elbow to your knee. Only allow the leg to dip as low as imprint can be maintained and keep the movement fluid – in other words, don't stop in the middle.

REGRESSIONS:

If you are struggling with the choreography, keep your feet on the mat and practise the upper body section first. Then practise just the leg section. Once they individually become second nature, you can combine the two.

PROGRESSIONS:

If you are strong, try to keep the pelvis in neutral rather than imprint. If you wish to challenge your core further, as you inhale and come through centre reach the arms long overhead before bringing them back behind your head as you rotate.

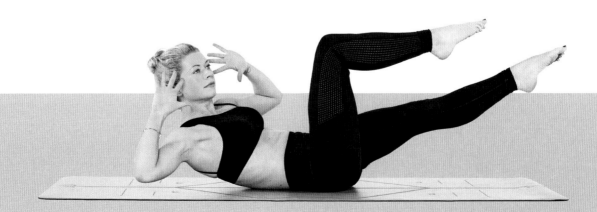

SCISSORS

This exercise feels like the most amazing stretch for the hamstrings while it also works to strengthen and lengthen the hip flexors. We are in thoracic flexion throughout so it will challenge your abdominal endurance, and you will be working hard (using your obliques) not to sway the pelvis from side to side. As with all the abdominal exercises, try not to create tension in the face or neck – keep all the effort in the tummy.

TARGET MUSCLES:

Transversus Abdominis *(to support the lumbar spine and pelvis)* | Pelvic Floor | Rectus Abdominis and Obliques *(to create thoracic flexion)* | Hip Flexors *(as the legs move)* | Obliques and Multifidus *(which work together to prevent rotation and rocking of the pelvis)*

REPS:

8–12

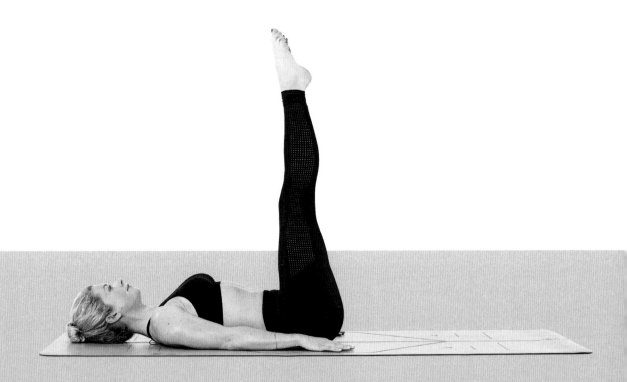

TECHNIQUE:

Start by lying on your back with your knees bent and feet on the floor, arms long by your sides. Imprint your spine and take your left leg into tabletop followed by your right before straightening the legs up to ceiling. Inhale to lengthen the back of the neck slightly and as you exhale contract the abdominals to flex your upper back and lift your head and shoulders away from the mat, reaching your hands up to your ankles. Inhale and as you exhale, for two counts, lower your left leg down towards the floor (keeping it straight) and reach your hands up towards your right ankle. Inhale to switch the legs at a half-way point and as you exhale, for two counts, reach the right leg away from the body and towards the floor, lifting your left leg back up towards the ceiling and reaching your hands up towards your left ankle. Complete all your reps before inhaling to reach both legs up and exhaling to lower your head back down and rest.

TEACHING POINTS:

As you lower your leg towards the ground, you should be sensing the feeling of lengthening out that leg. Imagine someone has grabbed your toes and is pulling your leg away from you slightly. There are two counts on the exhale for good reason: the first count is to lower the leg and the second is to reach even further. You are trying to extend/open your hip, but aim to keep the movement smooth. As you reach for your ankle, don't hold onto it for dear life – simply touch it.

REGRESSIONS:

If you have tight hamstrings and struggle to straighten your legs, feel free to have a slight bend at the knee and work on stretching your hamstrings separately. You can also practise the leg movement with your head and shoulders staying on the mat (make sure you keep imprint) to get used to the choreography and breath pattern.

PROGRESSIONS:

If you are strong, you can do this exercise with a neutral pelvis. If you would like to challenge your abdominals further, you can take your hands behind your head or straighten your arms out overhead to make them a longer, heavier lever.

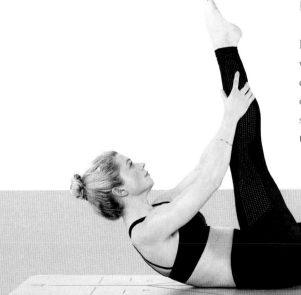

MERMAID PLANK

I'm not a fan of regular planks. You know – the ones where you are resting on your hands and trying to create a line, only for your lower back or shoulders to start aching and your body to shake uncontrollably. There is definitely a place for static plank holds but I really do prefer planks that require flow and movement, and side planks are incredible at building up muscles that protect our bodies in day-to-day activities. In this exercise we are taking the body into a movement it does very rarely in the day – everything is very forwards and backwards normally, but here we have side bending instead.

TARGET MUSCLES:
Scapula Stabilisers *(especially the serratus anterior, for the weight-bearing arm)* | Obliques *(to create lateral flexion and also to maintain a neutral lumbar spine with the help of the Multifidus)* | Adductors *(to press the legs together)* and Abductors *(to press away from the floor)* | Transversus Abdominis *(to support the lumbar spine and pelvis)* | Pelvic Floor | Hip Extensors

REPS:
4–6 on each side

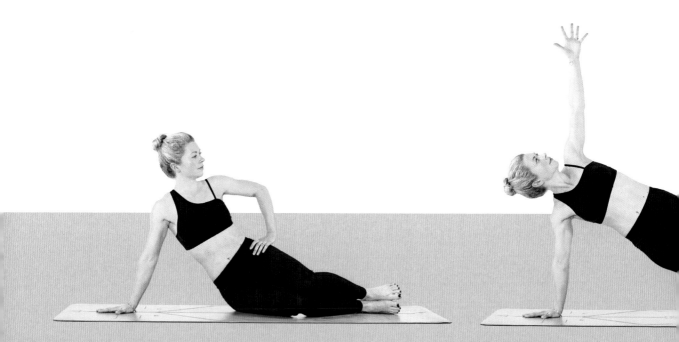

TECHNIQUE:

Start by sitting on your right hip, facing the side of your mat with your legs in line with your body. Have your feet stacked and your knees slightly bent. The weight should be on your right hand, which should be in line with your body and underneath your right shoulder. Your left hand is by your left side. Make sure you have a nice neutral pelvis. On your inhale, press your legs together and into the floor to lift the hips while straightening your legs and pressing into the floor – you should now be in a diagonal line (side plank) with your left arm lifted up to the ceiling. On your exhale, lift your hips up even higher, creating a side bend in the body, the shape of a crescent moon. On your next inhale, lower back to your side plank and on the exhale lower all the way back to your start position. Repeat all your reps on this side before switching over to your left side.

TEACHING POINTS:

This exercise passes from a neutral, straight spine on the side plank to lateral flexion (side bending) at the top. The lateral flexion is an important element and if you are able to look in a mirror you will know whether you have achieved it. Try not to sink into the supporting arm – feel as if you are pushing the floor away from you. Engage the glutes to maintain a neutral pelvis and press the inner thighs together. Keep the hips stacked so there is no rotation of the pelvis and keep the abdominals engaged.

REGRESSIONS:

Often it is getting the side bend into this exercise that is hard, so break it into two moves. First develop your side plank, then your side bend separately. Then combine the two moves into one. You can also try this with bent knees that stay on the ground, so you are a straight line from knee to head rather than feet to head.

PROGRESSIONS:

The slower we do this exercise, the more endurance is required from the muscles. If we add extra breaths into the exercise, we can slow it down. When you hit your side plank, stay still for a full breath before moving to the side bend. Then, when in the side bend, add in another full breath. Add in another breath on the side plank and then come down.

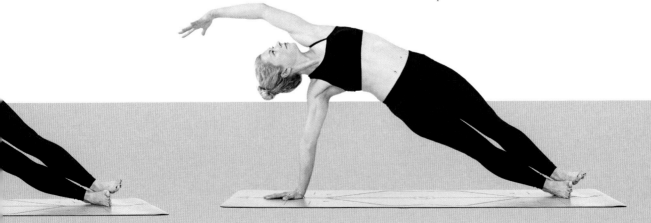

SWIMMING

Swimming is a great exercise for those who are kyphotic or have weak back extensors. It strengthens the erector spinae, which is a powerful postural muscle and is recruited especially by the thoracic spine here. Be careful not to lift too high as that will encourage the lumbar extensors to get involved, which we don't want. Imagine being long and low rather than looking like a banana.

TARGET MUSCLES:

Erector Spinae *(to extend the thoracic spine)* | Transversus Abdominis *(to support the lumbar spine and pelvis)* | Obliques and Multifidus *(to prevent the pelvis rocking from side to side)* | Obliques *(to prevent overextension of the lumbar spine)* | Gluteus and Hamstrings *(to lift the legs and extend the hips)* | Deltoids *(to lift the arms)* | Scapular Stabilisers *(to maintain neutral scapulae)*

REPS:

4–5 rounds

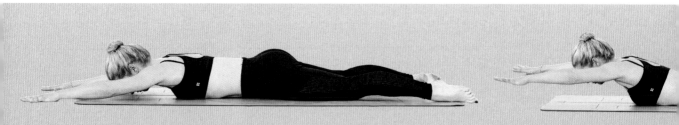

TECHNIQUE:

Start by lying on your tummy with your legs straight, parallel and hip-distance apart with toes pointed. Your arms should be overhead and resting on the ground, shoulder distance apart with palms down. Inhale and then as you exhale, keeping a neutral pelvis, lift and lengthen as much of the spine as you can, lifting the arms and legs away from the mat. Inhale for five counts, and lift one arm and the opposite leg higher, switching the limbs on every 'count'. It should look like you are swimming underwater. Exhale for five counts, continuing the movement. That is one 'round'. Perform 4–5 rounds (stop if you feel tension in your lower back). Once your rounds are complete, inhale to hold and exhale to lower your body back to the mat with control.

TEACHING POINTS:

This exercise is designed to strengthen the upper back. If we come up too high, we risk the effort coming from the lower back. Try to imagine that someone is pulling on your fingers and your toes, stretching you out. Try to keep the movement fluid and smooth, not too ballistic, and remember to breathe. Make sure the shoulder blades don't creep up to your ears too much.

REGRESSIONS:

It is usually the choreography on this exercise that people struggle with. It's quite tricky to get the opposite arm and leg coordinated so don't worry if you struggle with this. Instead keep the body on the ground (don't lift the chest off the floor) and on your exhale lift the arm and opposite leg off the floor and on the inhale lower them back to the ground. Then repeat on the other arm and leg. Eventually you will be able to speed this up and perfect the coordination.

PROGRESSIONS:

Go a little faster and try to do two movements on each count. This will further challenge your stability, coordination and endurance. As before, be careful not to wobble from side to side.

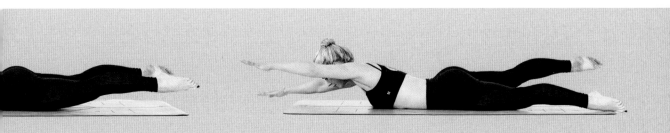

KYPHOSIS CORRECTOR

This exercise works the muscles of the upper back and helps to reduce postural issues. It's a great exercise for those who have shoulders that have collapsed forwards as it works the middle and lower trapezius muscles, which help to keep the shoulder blades where they belong. On the lift phase of the exercise, we are working the back extensors, which help you to sit and stand up straight and can often be weak. As with the Swimming exercise, stay low and long – don't force yourself to go too high.

TARGET MUSCLES:
Scapula Retractors *(to draw the shoulder blades together and down)* | Erector Spinae *(in the mid-back, to lift the spine)* | Obliques and Hip Extensors *(to keep the pelvis in neutral)* | Transversus Abdominis *(to support the lumbar spine and pelvis)* | Pelvic Floor

REPS:
4–6

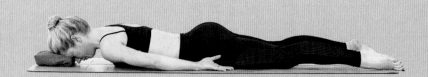
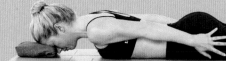

TECHNIQUE:

Start by lying on your front with a neutral pelvis, your arms straight and relaxed by your sides, legs straight and hip-distance apart. Your shoulders should be relatively relaxed, which will usually mean they fall forwards slightly due to gravity. On your inhale, draw your shoulder blades together enough to create a neutral shoulder blade position and open the front of the shoulders. On your exhale, lengthen out the spine, lifting the upper body very slightly away from the floor and reach your fingers back towards your toes. Inhale to hold, reaching the head forwards. On the exhale, slowly lower back to the start position with control. Repeat.

TEACHING POINTS:

The lift you create in your upper back should be very slight – we want thoracic extension, not lumbar. The pelvis should stay nice and neutral. Imagine drawing your shoulder blades down into a V position and opening up the collarbone. The legs should not leave the floor on this exercise.

REGRESSIONS:

Take the lifting of the spine out of the exercise and only focus on the shoulder blades moving. This will enable you to focus on the trapezius muscles and shoulder placement.

PROGRESSIONS:

Take your hands in front of your forehead, like a little pillow, and when you lift keep the hands against your skin. This will make you a heavier lever to lift and will be more effort for the back extensors. Make sure you still maintain a neutral pelvis and activate the muscles between the shoulder blades.

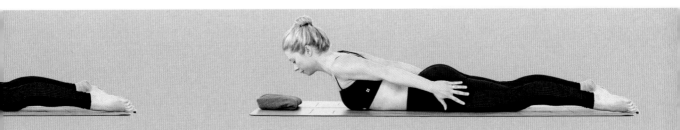

HIP TWIST

I really like this exercise as it combines so many muscles all into one tough, versatile exercise. If you have been practising The Model Method for a while now, this exercise will be a great test of your strength and stability. If you find you are moving your hips a lot, you are missing the essence of the exercise – I want you to stay steady and stable.

TARGET MUSCLES:

Rhomboids, Middle and Lower Trapezius, Latissimus Dorsi and Serratus Anterior *(to support the shoulder blades and prevent sinking into the arms)* | Hip Flexors *(to lift and lower the legs)* | Rectus Abdominis and Obliques *(to create lumbar flexion)* | Obliques *(to stop over-rotation of the pelvis)* | Pelvic Floor | Transversus Abdominis *(to support the lumbar spine and pelvis)*

REPS:

4–6 reps in each direction

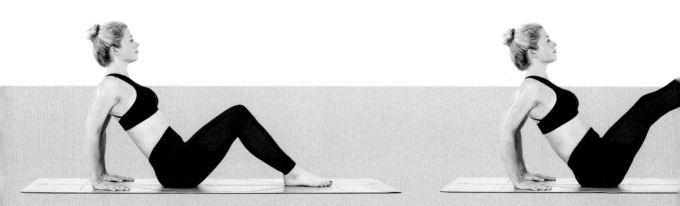

TECHNIQUE:

Start by sitting on the floor with your knees bent and feet on the floor. Flex your lower back by tucking your pelvis slightly back and leaning back, and reaching your arms behind you, palms on the floor, fingers pointing forwards. Now you want your upper back to be long while your lower back is tucked under, almost like you are making the letter J with your spine. Lift and straighten your legs up towards the ceiling as high as you can, keeping them together, while maintaining your position. Engage the core and inhale. As you exhale begin to circle your legs in a clockwise direction, keeping them together and straight and your pelvis still. As you inhale, complete the circle and come back to your start position. On your exhale, take your legs anti-clockwise and again as you inhale bring them back up the other side. Alternate the direction on each circle.

TEACHING POINTS:

Ensure you are not sinking into your arms – engage the muscles around the shoulder blades and keep the chest wide. Imagine you are almost showing off your chest. Maintain the lift through the thoracic spine and don't hunch. Try to allow the hip flexors to lengthen as the legs lower – don't let your pelvis go with them. Engage the core muscles to stabilise the pelvis but don't create tension in the face and neck.

REGRESSIONS:

If you have tight shoulders (especially if they hunch forwards), it might be difficult for you to rest on your hands, so lowering yourself down onto your forearms/elbows may help. It also takes the pressure off the hip flexors a little. If you have tight hamstrings, you can bend your knees a little, which will be more comfortable and give you a better range of movement.

PROGRESSIONS:

Going a little slower and drawing larger circles will make this exercise more challenging, but try to focus on keeping the steadiest of hips during the movement.

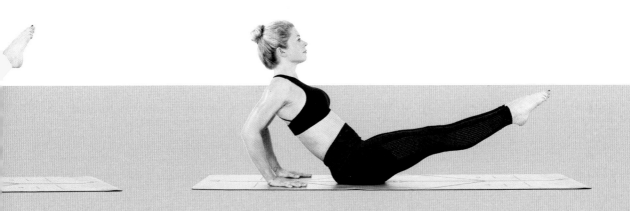

SINGLE-ARM PUSH-UP

This exercise is great for the triceps, pecs and scapula stabilisers as you work to steady the shoulder blade. It may feel a little strange at first but it is really functional. Ensure you are pressing your weight through your arm and not cheating by using your core. Almost imagine you are a dead weight as you push up. This is a great alternative to a regular press up if you struggle to hold your plank. There is very little pressure on the spine in this version and it can feel easier too.

TARGET MUSCLES:

Pectoralis Major and Anterior Deltoid *(to press away from the ground)* | Tricep *(to extend/straighten the elbow)* | Scapula Stabilisers *(to support the shoulder blade)* | Rotator Cuff and Latissimus *(to lift)*

REPS:

6–8 on each arm

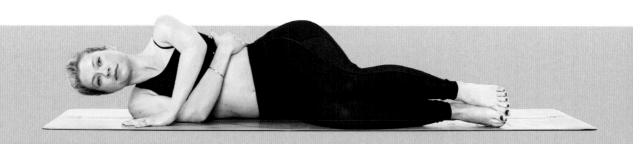

TECHNIQUE:

Start by lying on your right-hand side with your knees bent to tabletop on the floor in front of you. Your right arm should be wrapped around yourself like you are giving yourself a hug and your left hand should be on the floor just in front of your right shoulder (your elbow will be bent). Your core should be engaged and your spine in neutral – feel free to put a pillow or block under your head if it's more comfortable. Inhale and as you exhale press into your left hand to press your upper body away from the ground until your arm is straight. Try to keep your legs and bum on the ground. On your inhale, with control, slowly lower your body back to the start position. Repeat all reps on this side before switching over to lie on your left-hand side.

TEACHING POINTS:

Keep the core engaged as you push yourself up so that you retain a neutral spine – you should have created a diagonal line from hip to ear at the top of the push up. Try to keep your shoulder blade steady during the move and don't allow the shoulders to crunch up towards the ears. Come down with control – no collapsing back down.

REGRESSIONS:

If the struggle is completely straightening the arm here, reduce your range of movement. Maybe focus on just the initial press and come up just half way until you are able to push higher each time.

PROGRESSIONS:

Placing your hand further away from the body will put a greater emphasis on the pectorals as the tricep will have less work. Once you are competent at this exercise, however, you should move on to the Pilates Push-up (page 180), where you can practise full push-ups.

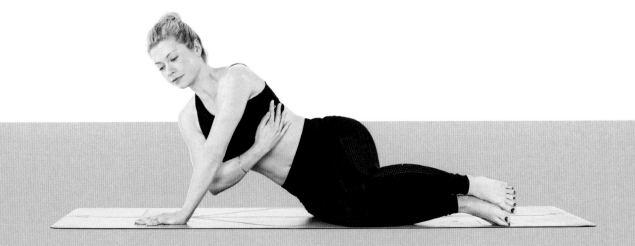

CACTUS

This exercise is great for those who have medially rotated arms (they've turned inwards) or hunched shoulders as it encourages endurance in the corresponding muscles. You might also feel a stretch in the muscles that are tight across your chest. Endurance of postural muscles is vital for long-term posture changes and, if you find this exercise tricky, chances are it's a good one for you!

TARGET MUSCLES:
External Rotators of the Arm | Deltoid and Supraspinatus *(to elevate the arm)* | Lower Trapezius *(to depress the scapula)*

REPS:
15–20

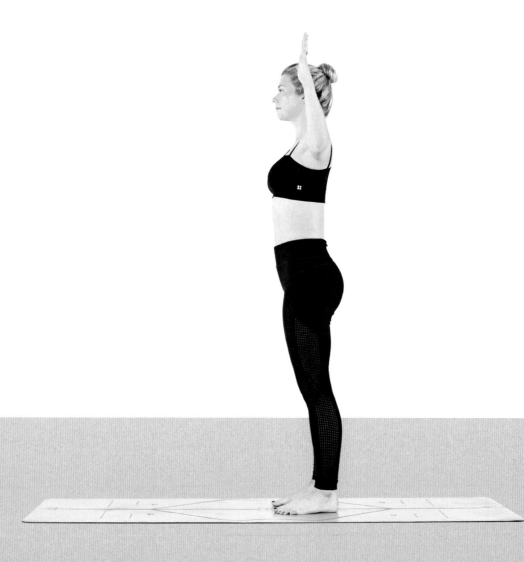

TECHNIQUE:

Stand with your back in neutral and resting against a wall (your feet may also be touching the wall but it will depend on how big your glutes are). Take your arms out to crucifix, along the wall and then bend the elbows to 90 degrees, again keeping them against the wall (you should look like a cactus). Make sure the shoulder blades are nice and neutral (not up by your ears). On your inhale, keep your elbows against the wall and rotate the arms so that your hands point down to the floor. Exhale to rotate them back to the start position. You are essentially rotating your arm in the shoulder socket. That is one rep.

TEACHING POINTS:

If you have a tight upper trapezius, which a lot of us do, be careful that the shoulder blades are not creeping up to your ears. Imagine the shoulder blades drawing down into a V-shape. Try to keep the elbows against the wall to ensure you keep width across your chest. Keep the elbows up as high as your shoulders.

REGRESSIONS:

If it is a struggle to keep your elbows against the wall, take them an inch away but ensure they stay there and don't deviate. If you are struggling to keep the shoulder blades down during the exercise, start with the elbows below shoulder height, creating a W rather than a cactus shape with your arms.

PROGRESSIONS:

Hold some dumb-bells or bottles of water to increase the resistance. Try to increase the range of movement at the shoulder on each rep to encourage shoulder mobility.

LEG PULL PREP

This exercise is actually great for the whole body but I like the effect it has on stretching the chest and strengthening the arms. This is a reverse of the position so many of us are in each day. It opens the front of the body and our hip extensors work against gravity here to lift the hips. If you have tight shoulders it may feel tough at first, but again the best way to improve is to practise. If you have problems with your wrists, please do the regression version.

TARGET MUSCLES:

Transversus Abdominis *(to support the lumbar spine and pelvis)* | Obliques and Rectus Abdominis *(to maintain slight thoracic and lumbar flexion)* | Hip Extensors *(to elevate the hips)* | Scapula Stabilisers *(to maintain neutral shoulder blades)* | Latissimus Dorsi and Teres Major *(to support the weight through the arms)*

REPS:

6–8

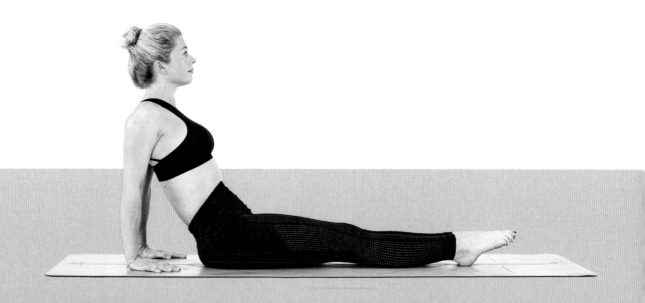

TECHNIQUE:

Start seated on a mat with your legs along the floor straight out in front of you and together. Your hands should be a few inches behind your bum with palms down and fingers pointing forwards. Make sure your collarbone is wide and your neck is in neutral. Inhale and as you exhale start to tuck the tailbone under slightly (into lumbar flexion) and start to lift the hips up towards the ceiling until you are one long line from ankles to ribs (keep slight thoracic flexion). As you inhale, slowly begin to lower back down, uncurling into a neutral spine at the bottom. Repeat.

TEACHING POINTS:

Keep your eyeline forwards throughout and don't allow your head to fall back at the top. Engage the core throughout and think about the shape your spine is making: you shouldn't look like the letter n at the top – you should look more like an opened out letter u. Don't sink into the shoulders and make sure the legs are active to take the pressure off the knees.

REGRESSIONS:

If this is a struggle for your shoulders, come down onto your forearms or elbows. This will also reduce the range of movement needed and may be more comfortable for some.

PROGRESSIONS:

Once you are at the top, without moving the rest of the body, lift your left foot off the floor an inch, then repeat with the right foot before slowly lowering the body back down.

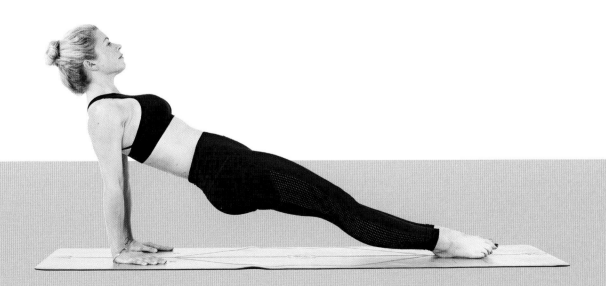

DUMB WAITER

This is another great exercise for those who sit hunched over their laptops all day. When we are in this position for extended periods, our arms medially rotate and we create a tight chest. This exercise encourages external rotation and wakes up the muscles in the upper back and around the shoulder blades. If you have a resistance band, loop or even a belt, hold this in your hands to give greater resistance. Using a mirror is really helpful in this exercise to monitor technique.

TARGET MUSCLES:
External Rotators of the Shoulder *(to turn the arms out)*
Lower and Middle Trapezius and Rhomboids *(to stabilise the scapula)* | Erector Spinae *(to maintain a neutral spine)*

REPS:
10–16

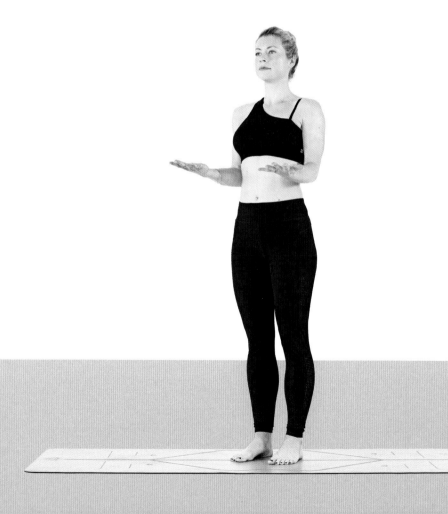

TECHNIQUE:

Stand with your feet hip-distance apart, spine and pelvis neutral and core gently engaged. Start by rolling your shoulders back and down and getting your shoulder blades into a neutral position. Bend your elbows forwards to 90 degrees with the palms facing up and imagine you have a plate on each hand. Make sure the tip of your elbow is underneath your shoulder joint. Inhale and as you exhale press your hands out to the sides, keeping your elbows against your body, as if you are passing your plates to people next to you. Inhale to bring them back to the start position. Repeat.

TEACHING POINTS:

Imagine you have a newspaper under each arm that you don't want to drop. This will prevent the elbow from moving away from under the shoulder joint. Also imagine that you are trying not to spill your spaghetti, so don't allow your hands to fall below elbow level. Try not to pinch the shoulder blades together as your arms open out – we want to keep the shoulder blades neutral. Keep your spine neutral throughout and your eyeline forwards.

REGRESSIONS:

If it is tiring maintaining a neutral spine while standing, try sitting down instead. Just ensure that you are still maintaining a neutral spine and are comfortable throughout.

PROGRESSIONS:

Adding a dumb-bell in each hand will challenge the biceps, or holding a resistance band will make it harder to separate your hands and will challenge the external rotators.

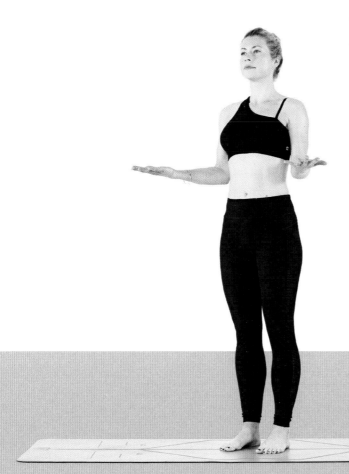

INCLINE PUSH-UP

This exercise challenges shoulder stability as you aim to perform a push-up with the arms above the head. There is a difference in weight distribution in this version compared to a standard push-up, and there is a greater emphasis on the pec muscles. If you are heavily kyphotic, you will be better doing the Pilates Push-up (page 180) instead as that recruits the triceps more.

TARGET MUSCLES:

Pectoralis Major and Triceps *(to complete the push up)* | Transversus Abdominis *(to support the lumbar spine and pelvis)* | Scapula Stabilisers *(to support the shoulder blades)* | Deltoids *(to support the shoulder)* | Muscles of the Spine *(support during the lowering phase)*

REPS:

4–6

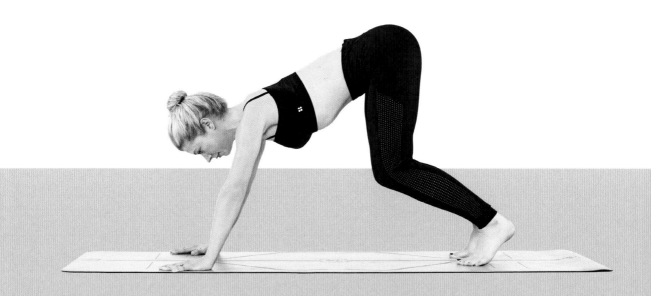

TECHNIQUE:

Start in a four-point kneeling position with your hands slightly wider than shoulder-width apart and your knees under your hips. Engage the core and lift your bum up to the ceiling, keeping a slight bend in the knees, placing the weight into your arms. Your arms should be slightly in front of your shoulders now, as if they are a little overhead. As you inhale, bend your elbows out to the sides of the room, carefully lowering your forehead towards the floor. Exhale to straighten your elbows and push yourself back up.

TEACHING POINTS:

Make sure you are moving slowly and with control, increasing the range of movement gradually so you don't end up face-planting the floor. Keep your abdominals engaged and the spine neutral – bend your knees more if this is a struggle. Your elbows should point out to the sides but watch the shoulder blades aren't creeping up to your ears.

REGRESSIONS:

Keep the knees down on the floor. You can still have your arms slightly forwards of your body by walking the hands forwards, but start on your knees until you're strong enough to build up.

PROGRESSIONS:

The more you straighten your legs and the higher your bottom, the more weight you place in your arms. Experiment with your placement to find a position that is challenging but safe for you.

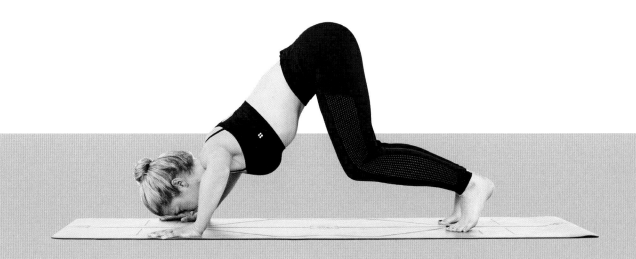

PILATES PUSH-UP

This exercise always goes at the end of a Pilates workout and I feel it's a really great way to end a session as it includes a roll down plus a test of your strength. Many people are able to do push-ups – however, performing them correctly is tough. We need very good control of our shoulder blades to do them properly and they should not be fast or ballistic. Take your time, build up your strength with the other arm exercises in The Model Method and even if you are normally really confident with push-ups try to take your time on these.

TARGET MUSCLES:

Transversus Abdominis *(to support the lumbar spine and pelvis)*
Pelvic Floor | Rectus Abdominis and Obliques *(to hold a neutral pelvis)* | Hip Extensors *(to maintain the plank position)* |
Scapula Stabilisers *(to support the shoulder blades)* | Triceps and Pectoralis Major *(to perform the push up)* | Rhomboids and Mid and Lower Trapezius | Back Extensors

REPS:

2–4 rounds

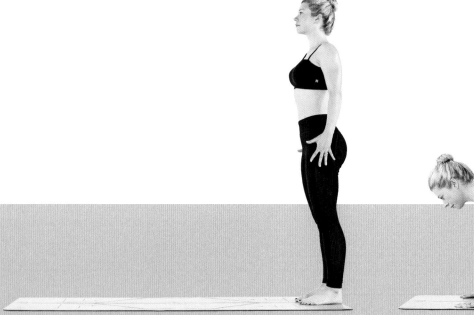
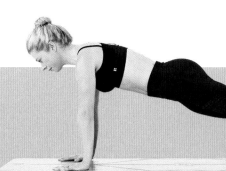

TECHNIQUE:

Start by standing at the end of your mat (facing the mat) with your legs together, a neutral pelvis and spine, and your arms by your sides. On your next inhale, begin to roll forwards and down through your spine one vertebra at a time, drawing your hands towards the floor, keeping the weight in the middle of your feet. As you exhale, taking four counts, start to walk your hands out along the mat until you reach a plank position (try not to rock from side to side as you do so). Inhale, for three counts, and bend the elbows backwards diagonally, lowering your body towards the floor. Exhale to straighten your arms and come back to your plank. Repeat for three push ups in total. Inhale and over four counts walk your hands back towards your feet, keeping your spine flexed rather than straight. Exhale and slowly rebuild the spine back up one vertebra at a time until you reach your start position. That is one round.

TEACHING POINTS:

Make sure that as you roll down and back up you do so with a flexed/rounded spine, not a straight one. You are trying to articulate your spine with control. When you lower down into your push-up, ensure your pelvis stays neutral and that you are not dipping through your lower back. Keep your neck in line with the spine throughout – no craning your head backwards.

REGRESSIONS:

Practise your push-ups in a half plank position (with knees on the floor). As you bend the elbows, focus on the line you are drawing from knees to shoulders and ensure it stays neutral. Once you are strong enough, aim for a full plank position.

PROGRESSIONS:

Try the exercise with one leg extended behind you (i.e. standing on one leg). As you roll down, elevate your back leg, similarly to the Arabesque Deadlift, and keep your foot off the floor during the push up. This will require you to recruit your core more to prevent rotation of the pelvis.

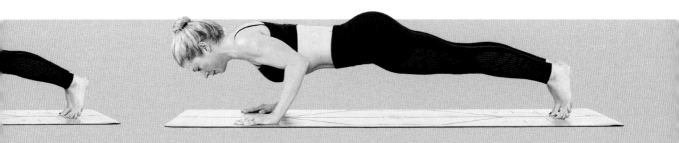

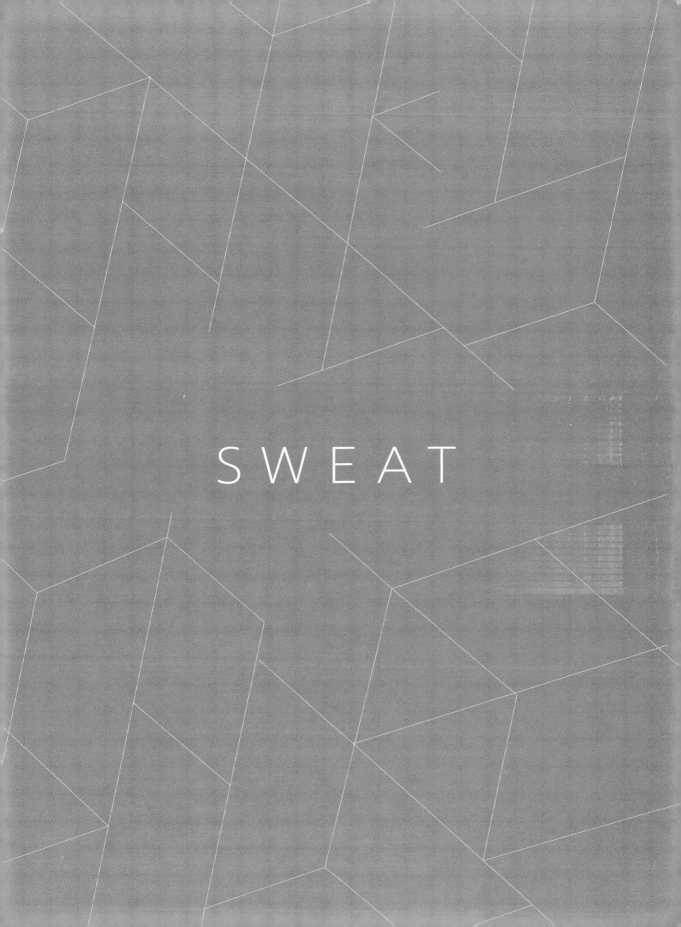

SWEAT

SWEAT

It's no secret that exercise plays an important role in health management. There are real health benefits to an active lifestyle and conversely there are risks for those who are inactive. Studies have found that increasing physical activity reduces mortality levels, [17] and this is true no matter your BMI or waist circumference. There are many reasons to move your body more, and this does not mean an hour of pounding the treadmill or jumping around in an aerobics class. This can be as simple as walking your dog, doing the housework or dancing around your bedroom. Anything that gets the heart pumping and your muscles working will have a positive effect on your health and happiness. You can't rely on a healthy diet alone to improve your health, and learning to love exercise is one of the kindest things you can do for your body. Our bodies were designed to run, jump, hop, bend and bounce, and we have incredible energy systems in place to allow us to do so. The old adage of 'if you don't use it you'll lose it' is true for strength and cardiovascular ability. Short, regular blasts of exercise are far more beneficial than irregular, never-ending sessions at the gym.

Just as everyone's dietary requirements are different, everyone's bodies are different and the type of exercise you enjoy or need will vary. For many years I found yoga slow and a little boring, favouring fast spin classes or noisy gyms. This was great for a period of time in which I had lots of energy to burn and I was motivated by speed and power workouts. Now, with a hectic schedule and a demanding business, I really do love adding a yoga class into my weekly routine and rely on the mental health benefits it brings. Make sure that whatever method of moving your body you choose, you enjoy it. Life is too short to be slogging away at a spin class, hating life, if you could spend that hour loving your body (and your workout) at a Pilates studio (or vice versa).

The biggest impact on my physical fitness, however, has come from high-intensity interval training (HIIT), which I began researching when I was creating The Model Method. I wanted to find something that would improve my clients' cardiovascular fitness, reduce any levels of unhealthy visceral fat and empower them to work hard and enjoy their workouts. I also needed to make sure that it didn't eat too much into their day or their sessions with me as that would make them far less likely to commit to it in the long run. HIIT seemed to tick all the boxes and I have seen it change women's health, confidence and fitness, time and time again. My clients have improved their functional fitness, lowered their body-fat levels (in those whose body-fat levels were medically seen as high), grown to enjoy exercise and felt more confident in their abilities. They are not afraid of trying out their local climbing wall, or joining netball teams, or even signing up for marathons. They are empowered, physically and mentally strong, and motivated to look after their bodies. I hope that this will pass on to you too.

WHAT HAPPENS TO OUR BODIES WHEN WE EXERCISE?

Wow, where to start? The body is quite possibly the most amazing, most versatile and most perfect machine that exists. While we are completely oblivious to its inner goings-on, our body is working at full pelt to ensure that we are safe, functional and adapting to the environment around us. If we could look inside ourselves, we would see millions of chemical reactions, processes and feedback mechanisms working tirelessly to create this incredible body we all own. I like to remind clients of this when they start talking negatively about their body. It is all well and good to say 'I stopped going to spinning because my thighs were getting bigger' (if I had £1 for every time I've heard that . . .) but that's effectively a massive 'screw you' to your body, which didn't actually make you 'bigger' but rather adapted its lung size, heart strength and muscle shape in thanks for you taking part in cardiovascular fitness. It's your body that's doing all the hard work and making the changes necessary for exercise to be more enjoyable and less painful – don't give up just as the effects start to show. Thank your body for being so adaptable that you were able to finish a spin class.

I would therefore like you all to know some of the main processes that are taking place while you exercise. Knowledge is power, and if we are to really learn what our bodies need we must first learn how they work.

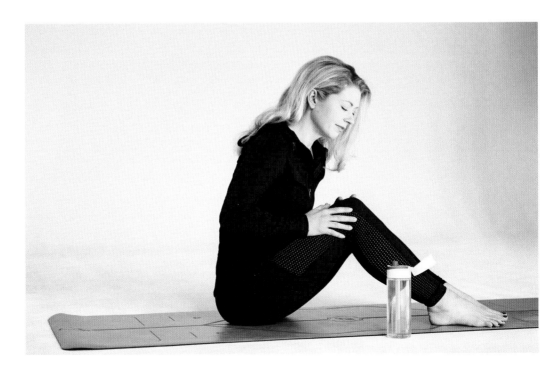

OUR BREATH PATTERN CHANGES

When we inhale, we are, in normal circumstances, breathing in a combination of nitrogen, oxygen, carbon dioxide and a very small amount (1 per cent) of other gases. The muscles in our chest work to lift the ribcage, expand the lungs and encourage air to flow in from the environment. Inside the lungs, gaseous exchange takes place whereby oxygen (which we really want in our bodies) is drawn out of the lungs and into the blood stream and carbon dioxide (which we don't want in our bodies any more) is passed from the blood stream back into the lungs. On an exhale, our ribcage is pulled back down and the air (now with more carbon dioxide and less oxygen) is sent back out into the environment.

The gaseous exchange that takes place in our lungs is an incredible way of harnessing the materials our body needs (oxygen) and getting rid of waste we do not need (carbon dioxide) during breathing. The lungs interact with the blood as it makes its way around the body. As deoxygenated blood goes through the lungs, it drops off waste carbon dioxide and collects oxygen to take to the heart. The heart then sends these oxygenated blood cells around the body, where they can hand their oxygen off to where it's needed and then head back to the lungs for more oxygen again. This journey is cyclical, as the blood moves from the lungs to the heart to the body to the heart and then back again to the lungs. The red blood cells are acting as delivery drivers for oxygen and the blood is a removal van for carbon dioxide.

When we exercise, there is a greater demand for oxygen in the muscle cells (which you will learn more about soon). We need oxygen to create energy, and carbon dioxide is the waste product created in this process. Our breath rate increases when we exercise to enable more oxygen to be taken into the body and more carbon dioxide to be breathed out.

HOMEOSTASIS KEEPS US 'NORMAL'

I really enjoy a warm house. If it's chilly I'll put the fire on. Too hot and I'll open the windows. However, if I used my boiler's thermostat, the temperature of my home would be regulated at just the right temperature for me. This is the equivalent of my home's 'homeostasis'. Our bodies like things a certain way too. They know that there is an optimum internal environment that works best for us. They like the temperature just right (37 degrees), the blood sugar to be controlled, the water content of the body to be maintained and so on. The body has powerful feedback mechanisms that let it know if something is not quite right, and these trigger hormones in the body to bring it back to homeostasis. It's very clever and very intuitive, and it plays an important role in exercise. So let's see how the body adapts to exercise and what actually happens when we train our bodies.

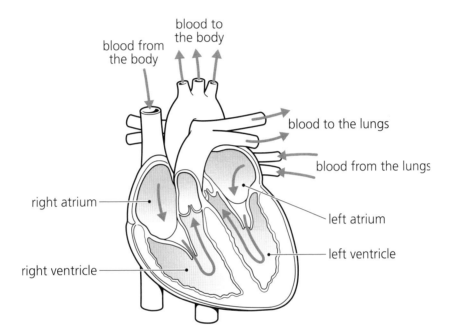

blood to
the body

blood from
the body

blood to the lungs

blood from the lungs

right atrium

left atrium

left ventricle

right ventricle

The heart is broken down into four chambers. Atria collects blood from the body while ventricles pump the blood away from the heart. The heart ensures blood moves around the body. If we imagine how many veins, capillaries and arteries there are in our body and how vast our bodies are, we can see why the heart has a huge role. If we didn't have the heart, our blood would simply pool down to our feet and very little would reach the brain (thanks, gravity).

It would also mean blood wouldn't circulate around the body – but our blood is a vital transport mechanism for oxygen, carbon dioxide, hormones, nutrients and waste. Blood makes its way back to the heart (via the pulmonary veins) when it has collected oxygen from the lungs. It's ready and raring to go to pass its package of oxygen, hormones, etc. on to the rest of the body. The heart is a muscle, but it's a cardiac muscle, which is a different type from the muscles we use to move our bodies. Part of this difference is that it contracts completely involuntarily (we don't have to sit and think 'OK, heart, beat now'). As the heart contracts, the oxygenated blood flows, under high pressure, to the rest of the body.

This blood makes its way around the whole body (e.g. some goes to the upper body, some to the lower, some to your digestive system and some to your liver). Once the blood is done passing on all its oxygen to your organs and muscles (which will be explained later), it needs to make its way back to the lungs for some more oxygen (and to drop off its carbon dioxide). The veins of the body, which are large and contain valves that prevent blood flowing backwards, carry the now deoxygenated blood from the body back to the heart.

As before, the heart uses a big push to send the blood out to the lungs, where it performs gaseous exchange and collects more oxygen. The whole process repeats itself as the blood heads back to the heart to be sent around the body again. It typically all works in unison and the process keeps our bodies moving, our muscles functioning and our brains alive.

When we exercise, our muscles require oxygenated blood at a much faster rate than at rest. This is why our heart rate increases during exercise as it works harder to send more blood to the muscles. Remember that our heart is a muscle and muscles can be strengthened. When we exercise, we are not only strengthening our superficial muscles, such as the abdominals – we are also strengthening our heart.

As your heart gets stronger, it is able to push more blood out around the body on each beat (this is called stroke volume). If we are able to push more blood out on each pump, our heart doesn't have to pump as often to have the same effect. This is seen in those who are fit as a low resting heart rate. Their hearts are so efficient at pumping blood around the body that they don't have to beat as fast. This is a fantastic reason to carry out exercise that gets the heart beating faster (cardiovascular exercise) and strengthens your heart.

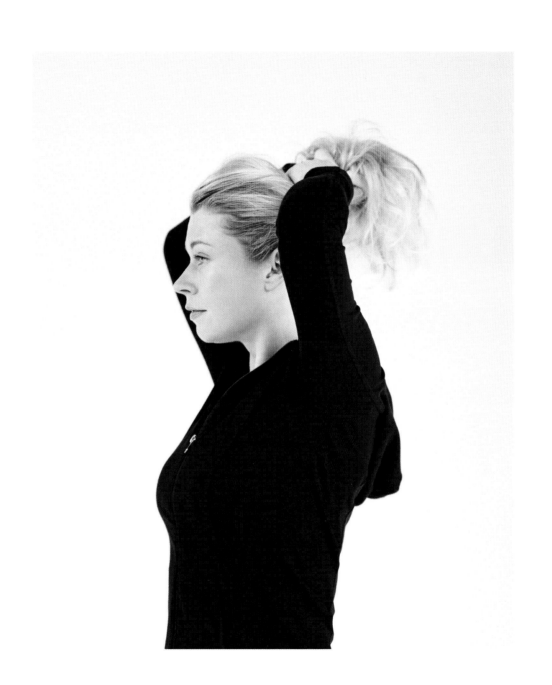

Our bodies work in a very similar way to a car. With a car, we put fuel in and we get mileage out. In our bodies, what we eat is broken down into small energy units and either stored for later (in adipose tissue, in the liver, in our muscles or in other cells) or excreted. Our body tries to keep as much energy from our food as possible in case of emergency (such as famine, a tiger chasing us, a particularly tough winter, etc.). When we exercise, we tap into those energy reserves – however, unlike a car, the body has a variety of fuelling methods to choose from and it switches between them depending on the type of exercise undertaken.

Adenosine triphosphate (ATP) is the name of our energy currency (our petrol). It is stored in cells around the body ready to be used when needed and is incredibly versatile. When broken down, ATP becomes adenosine diphosphate (ADP) and energy is released. The more intense the exercise, the more ATP we need. Because ATP is such a vital source of energy, we are able to recycle it and the body converts ADP back to ATP (by adding a phosphate back again) to keep a constant supply.

When we carry out steady, low-intensity exercise, such as a 30 minute jog, glucose in our body is broken down and provides us with ATP for energy. The waste products of this reaction are carbon dioxide (which is then exhaled in our breath) and water. This reaction is called 'aerobic respiration' and requires a constant supply of oxygen to the muscles to take place. It is slow (so wouldn't allow you to run too fast) but can last for long periods of time. It is used during most exercise formats that last over two minutes as the alternative (anaerobic respiration) is only suitable for short bursts of exercise. When our stores of glucose are depleted, our body turns first to fat to aid ATP production, and in extreme circumstances it would then turn to protein.

When we start gearing up for 'exercise' (which could be anything from a spin class to running for the bus), it takes the heart and lungs a while to give your muscles the oxygen levels needed for aerobic respiration to take place. We instead use a process called 'anaerobic respiration', which gives us energy without oxygen. Now, the body only stores a small amount of ATP in the muscle cells, and this can fuel your exercise only for a very limited time. This would get us through the first three seconds of a 100-metre sprint. Then we'd have to start recycling that ATP using other substances in our cells.

But what happens if we need to run for longer? In a 200-metre race, our body would go through the same process as above and then turn to using glycogen instead (which our bodies store reserves of). Without oxygen in this reaction, our body would end up with a waste product called 'lactic acid' left behind. This would build up in our cells as our

200-metre sprint took place until eventually it would reach a level that would be painful and inhibit muscle contraction – in other words, we'd really want to stop or slow down. After this point, we'd no longer work at the same level any more and would need to slow down slightly, or stop, and let aerobic respiration take over.

So, if we were to decide to run a marathon, we would need to use the aerobic system to be able to complete the race. The body is incredible in allowing us to keep running for such long periods of time, and again this is due to the storage of fuel from our diets. The body first breaks down glucose, then fat, then protein and uses it efficiently for energy. We could not sprint a marathon, only jog it.

So we can see that different intensities of exercise prompt the body to use different energy systems. Aerobic respiration harnesses 19 times more energy than anaerobic but is much slower to initiate. When we perform HIIT, we use anaerobic respiration – and the benefits of this will be discussed soon.

WE INCREASE OUR BLOOD FLOW

During exercise, our body works hard to deliver oxygenated blood to the working muscles, as quickly as it can. I mentioned earlier that our heart rate speeds up to allow a quicker delivery of blood and to assist in the removal of carbon dioxide. Other methods are also used by the body to ensure a constant supply of oxygen to the muscles. When our muscles break down ATP, the by-products they give off stimulate the walls of the local blood vessels to dilate (expand) to allow more blood to pass through them. The brain also works to re-route blood that was meant for other areas (such as the kidneys or stomach) and send it to the working muscles instead. This is why it is not advisable to eat too close to a workout as your body will struggle to digest your meal while it's trying to exercise too. The blood that flows to the muscles not only brings goodies such as oxygen – it also helps to clear away waste products. So, the flow of blood around the body is of great importance in our endurance when we exercise.

When ATP is broken down to ADP, we generate energy but we also generate heat. This heat accumulates in the body and we can feel it. When our body senses we are heating up, as a method of homeostasis, the blood vessels that lie close to the skin dilate (expand), thus allowing the heat, carried in our blood, to escape through the skin. Our skin has a huge surface area and this is a really effective way of cooling down; it is also this very technique that gives us a red glow during exercise. To assist in this process, the brain tells our body to sweat and the evaporation of sweat from our bodies also works to cool us down.

EXCESS POST-EXERCISE OXYGEN CONSUMPTION

After exercise, you may find that your breath does not slow down straight away or that you are panting even once you have ceased your workout. This is our body's way of bringing about homeostasis and returning itself to the way it was before we started our workout (remember, your body likes normal). There is an increase in oxygen uptake during this time. This period of increased metabolism is called 'excess post-exercise oxygen consumption' (EPOC) and has various benefits to our health.

When we exercise, our bodies are working hard to draw as much oxygen to the muscles as possible by increasing our heart rate and our breathing rate. In this process, the breakdown of ATP to energy creates by-products, such as painful lactic acid, that require oxygen to break them down and remove them from the body or recycle them.

Once we have finished exercising, this is the perfect opportunity to do just that. We continue to have an increased breathing rate and our metabolism stays elevated somewhat so that we can get as much oxygen as possible to our muscles to flush out the by-products. We are trying to re-oxygenate our blood and refuel our energy systems. You can almost imagine EPOC as your body's way of clearing up after a house party before your parents get home (I haven't lived at home for 20 years but you get the picture). We continue in a state of increased metabolism while we carry on bringing the body back to homeostasis.

The benefits of EPOC are that it keeps your body working, and your metabolism increased, long after you cease your workout. This means that certain shorter workouts can have a similar effect on the body as a longer workout. However, the shorter workout must be of a high intensity (you guessed it – HIIT is the winner here). Increasing the intensity of a workout has been shown to increase the duration of EPOC,[18] and HIIT can therefore extend the duration of EPOC – and the benefits gained from it.

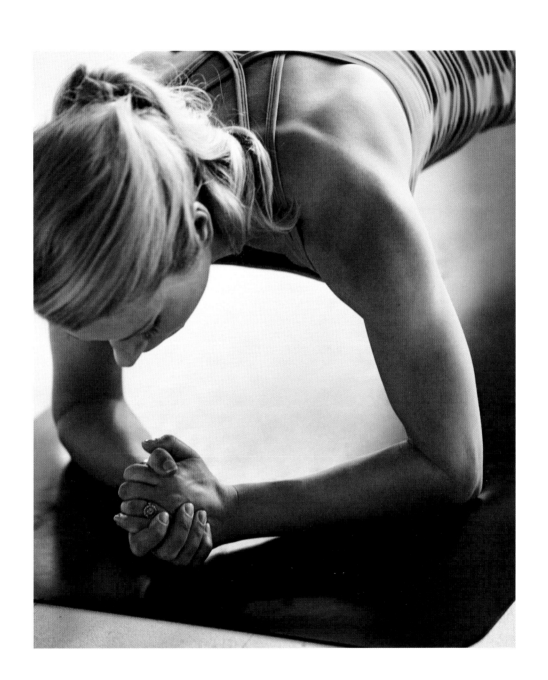

WHAT IS HIIT?

HIIT is an exercise method that incorporates short, high-intensity bursts of exercise with recovery periods at moderate to low intensity. This means you exercising at a pace that gets your heart rate up to 80–95 per cent of its maximum (I'll explain heart rates soon – see page 196), before allowing a rest period where it drops back down to around 40–50 per cent. The length of each high-intensity set can vary dramatically (there are lots of conflicting opinions on optimal set lengths), from 10 seconds to 8 minutes; however, it is most common for high-intensity periods to last between 30 seconds and 2 minutes. Recovery periods can also vary in length, as can the number of sets. However, most HIIT workouts last no more than 20–30 minutes, making them time efficient and easier to fit into your day than many other styles of exercise.

HIIT has grown in popularity over the years as research has supported the theory that HIIT can have the same benefits (and often more) as sustained, moderate-intensity cardiovascular exercise. This means that despite HIIT workouts taking less time, they are still as effective as other forms of cardiovascular exercise, with potentially even more benefits! It can feel really strange, if you are someone who is used to completing hour-long jogs or numerous lengths in the pool, to suddenly drop back to short, sharp workouts – but the science is really starting to back it up. Let's look at some of the main benefits.

REDUCTIONS IN SUBCUTANEOUS AND VISCERAL BODY FAT

Research into the effects of HIIT on body composition is still relatively new and there are many different forms HIIT can take. Many of the current studies have targeted young overweight individuals. This research has shown that HIIT can result in a significant reduction in subcutaneous and visceral body fat (remember that subcutaneous fat is the fat that lies directly under our skin whereas visceral fat is the fat around our organs).[19,20] Often, HIIT has been found to markedly outperform steady-state aerobic exercise with regard to fat reduction. This means that, despite the fact that we spend less time on our HIIT workouts and that we burn far fewer calories during HIIT training than in steady-state aerobic exercise (such as a 40-minute jog), we see far better results when it comes to the breakdown of body fat. If you think back to the Nourish chapter, visceral fat is linked to various health risks (in fact, visceral fat levels, compared to overall obesity, are more strongly associated with cardiovascular disease risk[21]). Any form of exercise that can reduce visceral fat levels is a winner in my book.

IMPROVEMENTS TO FITNESS LEVELS

HIIT has been found to improve both aerobic and anaerobic fitness.[21] 'VO2 max' is the name given to the maximum rate of oxygen consumption of an individual during exercise. It effectively shows us a person's aerobic fitness levels. Research has shown that HIIT can significantly improve our VO2 max levels.[22] Thus, despite being an anaerobic exercise, HIIT improves your aerobic fitness (as shown by your VO2 max). Studies also show increased anaerobic abilities in those who have completed a period of HIIT training.[23] Basically, HIIT improves our fitness levels in terms of both aerobic and anaerobic exercise. Our bodies adapt to use our oxygen intake better and HIIT brings about skeletal muscle adaptations.[19] If you are someone who enjoys aerobic exercise – such as long-distance running, swimming or team sports – then HIIT can help to improve your fitness in these areas.

IMPROVED INSULIN SENSITIVITY

Insulin is a hormone that is produced by the body when glucose is present. When we eat a meal containing carbohydrates, our blood-sugar levels rise and our body responds by producing insulin. The insulin in turn tells our cells to absorb the available glucose to be used later on. If we have more sugar in our blood stream than the cells can absorb, the insulin tells our liver to store it for later, and the liver can then release it into the bloodstream as and when it is needed. Those who are insulin resistant struggle to react to insulin's messages. The cells do not absorb the glucose and the sugar stays in the bloodstream. The body responds by secreting more insulin, but again this has no or little effect and our blood-sugar level remains high. This, as you might imagine, is not a good thing. HIIT has been shown to improve insulin sensitivity,[24, 25] which means the body responds better to insulin's messages.

There is a lot more to learn about HIIT and why it has the effects it does, but the research is incredibly promising. I personally have found that my body-fat levels have dropped since I added HIIT into my fitness regime, and studies show that, compared to endurance training, HIIT is better at fat oxidation.[26]

HEART RATE

When we talk about HIIT, we talk about our heart rate approaching a percentage, such as 80 per cent. But what does this number mean? This is actually describing the percentage of your maximum heart rate you are working at, at any one time. It is an indicator of how hard you (or more accurately your heart) are working. It is essential that you are working hard enough in your HIIT sessions to ensure you are targeting your anaerobic system.

So, first let's work out your maximum heart rate. To do so, use the equation for females below:

206 – (your age × 0.88) = maximum heart rate (in beats per minute)

Now, the number you have come out with is the maximum number of beats per minute (bpm) your heart should, in theory, go to. We use this maximum heart rate during HIIT. We might say, for example, that we need to get our heart rate up to 80 per cent of that maximum. So let's say your maximum heart rate is 180. This would mean that in your HIIT sessions you would need to aim for a heart rate of at least 144bpm (this is 80 per cent of 180). In my sessions, I use a heart rate monitor and I encourage my clients to do so too. A monitor can usually tell you either what your bpm is or what percentage of your maximum you are at. This is incredibly useful and it helps my clients to know when they are not working hard enough. These types of heart rate monitor usually give you a report at the end of your workout telling you how hard you worked on average during your session and how long your session was.

Wearing a heart rate monitor may not be feasible for you, so don't panic if you don't have one or prefer not to use one. You could in theory check your own heart rate at the end of a HIIT set to see what your bpm is. This would be quite time consuming but more accurate than guessing. However, I prefer to use a scale of 1–10 when I am without a heart rate monitor. I create a scale of exertion with 10 being the feeling that I am working as hard as physically possible and 1 being that I am doing nothing at all. During my HIIT sessions, I aim to work at the 9 out of 10 level. If you get used to checking in with how your body feels and where you are on that scale, you will be able to push yourself without the need of a monitor.

Whatever method you choose, I want you to be aiming for 80–90 per cent of your maximum heart rate during your high-intensity intervals and around 40–50 per cent of your maximum heart rate during your low-intensity intervals. We want the body to fluctuate from low to high heart rates throughout to allow recovery times in between each high-intensity set. The recommended timings for your sets can be found on page 199.

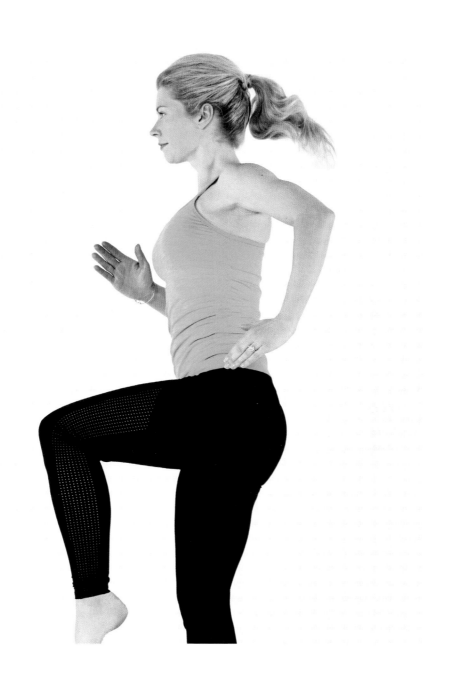

HIIT AND THE MODEL METHOD

The Model Method combines HIIT with Pilates. I strongly feel that HIIT is beneficial for building cardiovascular fitness and endurance and for promoting healthy levels of body fat. Combining it with Pilates covers your cardiovascular fitness while also taking care of your body's strength, flexibility and functionality. HIIT, despite being incredibly effective, feels tough. In The Model Method, you will practise your HIIT workouts three times per week, on alternating days, and will require no equipment except a yoga mat.

In HIIT, you are pushing your body out of its comfort zone and challenging your anaerobic system. You are also pushing your heart to work harder (and be strengthened in the process) and telling your body to function more effectively to help your muscles cope with the demand. For this reason, no matter what your fitness level, HIIT can feel really tough and it can occasionally be hard to motivate yourself. I know – I have been through the same journey myself. However, I do want to reassure you that it gets easier. The feelings you have after HIIT are of a real sense of achievement. You should feel empowered and controlled. It is as much about your mindset as it is your ability. You have two options: you can choose to think 'that was hard, I'm not doing that again' or you can choose to think 'that was tough, and I managed it, and my body is incredible for allowing me to do that. I know this will improve my fitness and I will get used to these feelings.' Please, please do try to keep your thoughts positive and proactive. You will gain so much for your efforts. The only way to get better at something is to practise it – doing nothing helps nobody.

YOUR SWEAT WORKOUT

In your Strengthen chapter, I showed you how to evaluate your body and its physical strengths and weaknesses. I gave you the option to choose which area(s) of your body you wanted to work on, and your exercises were listed in body areas to help you target just those areas.

In your sweat workout, the exercises are again split into body areas. However, here I want you to choose one exercise from each body area for each workout.

As we read earlier, when we work a muscle anaerobically, there is a build-up of lactic acid. This build-up is felt as a deep muscle burn but it also slows down muscle contraction. This slowing down forces us more towards aerobic respiration. If you choose exercises that work complementary muscle groups, it will allow you more chance of maintaining your momentum. For example, I may choose my first HIIT exercise to be Starbursts. This is from the Lower Body section. I will therefore need to choose one exercise from the Core section and one from the Upper Body section to complement the Starbursts.

During your sweat workouts, I want your high-intensity sets to alternate between each of these three exercise choices (lower body, core and upper body). An example is below.

Beginner level: Start with a warm-up of 90 seconds, then move on to the following:

Starburst	20 seconds
Rest	40 seconds
Half Burpee	20 seconds
Rest	40 seconds
Plank to Pike	20 seconds
Rest	40 seconds

This is one round (excluding the warm up, which you only do once). You will do five rounds followed by a cool down for 2 minutes. In total the workout time comes to 18.5 minutes.

The work-to-rest timings for different levels of fitness are below:

Beginner	work for 20 seconds, rest for 40 seconds	5–6 rounds
Intermediate	work for 30 seconds, rest for 60 seconds	4–5 rounds
Advanced	work for 40 seconds, rest for 80 seconds	4–5 rounds
Super-advanced	work for 45 seconds, rest for 60 seconds	4–5 rounds

A NOTE ON WARM-UPS

Completing a thorough warm-up before any activity is vital to prevent injury and facilitate movements. A warm-up is usually a low intensity version of the upcoming activity. In your sweat workouts you will be jumping, hopping and bouncing while getting your heart rate higher so your warm-up should include these types of movements. I have listed three to get you started but feel free to add your own. In the warm-up exercises listed you will be bending, squatting, rotating and jumping, and you should feel warmer, looser and ready to exercise. If you are feeling particularly stiff or sluggish please extend the length of your warm up.

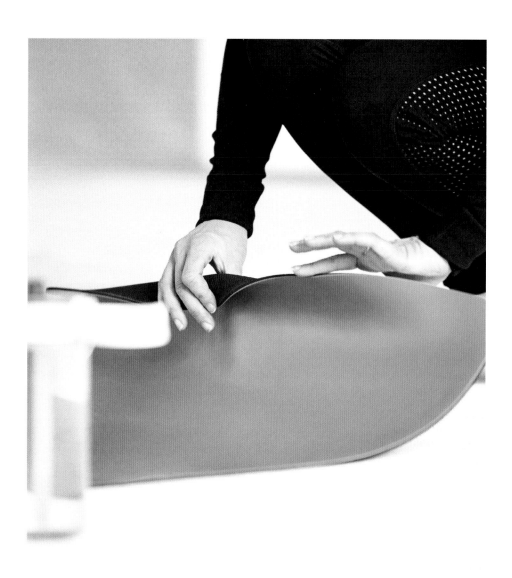

YOUR SWEAT EXERCISES

Do your HIIT exercises every other day (three days per week) for 20–30 minutes, on the days you are not practising your Pilates exercises. See pages 198–200 for how to incorporate the HIIT exercises into The Model Method plan.

WARM UP

Squat Rotations

High Knees

Jumping Jacks

LOWER BODY DOMINANT

Starbursts

Knee Pull

Skaters

Surfers

Floor to Ceiling

Kneel Up

Three-bounce Burpee

CORE DOMINANT

Half Burpee

Tombstones

Shoulder Taps

Walk the Plank

Plank Kick-through

Monkey Rope

Swing Planks

UPPER BODY DOMINANT

Plank to Pike

Triangle Push-up

Donkey Kicks

Push-up to Side Plank

Can Can

Monkey Walk

SQUAT ROTATIONS

Squat rotations will warm up the main, or global muscles of the legs while loosening up the muscles around the spine. Be careful that the exercise is not too ballistic and make it smooth and flowing.

TARGET MUSCLES:	TIME:
Glutes | Hamstrings | Quadriceps | Rotators of the Spine	30 seconds

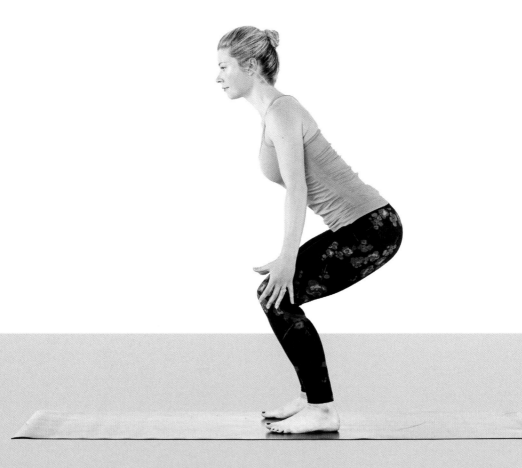

TECHNIQUE:

Stand with feet hip-distance apart and arms by your sides. Bend at the knees and hips, sitting into an imaginary chair. Stand up and as you do so rotate the upper body to one side and reach your arms up above your head, before returning the upper body to the centre. Repeat, alternating your rotations from side to side.

TEACHING POINTS:

Ensure you keep a neutral spine when squatting. No hunching. Push up through the heels as you stand. Try not to swing the arms and risk leaning back. Rotate from your waist upwards and be sure to keep your head in line with your spine.

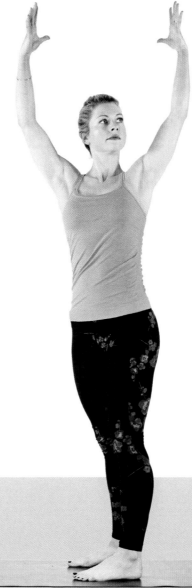

HIGH KNEES

High knees are a great way to lift the heart rate and prepare you for running and jumping. If you have tight hip flexors you may find they start to cramp, so reduce the range of movement when this happens.

TARGET MUSCLES:	TIME:
Hip Flexors | Glutes | Hamstrings | Quadriceps	30 seconds

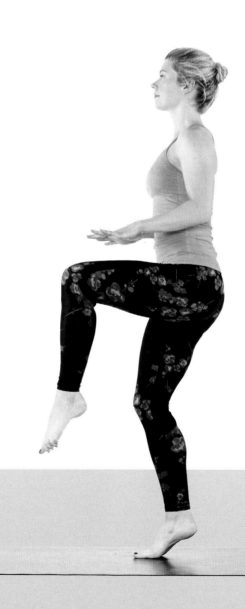

TECHNIQUE:

Begin by jogging on the spot. Start to pick up the pace and lift your knees higher and higher until they approach hip height. You can put your hands in line with your elbows and aim to tap your knees against your hands.

TEACHING POINTS:

You may have to lean back to counterbalance but ensure the core is engaged and there is no pain in the lower back.

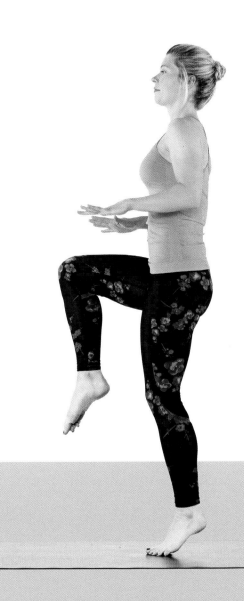

JUMPING JACKS

Jumping jacks are a great warm-up exercise as they involve the whole body and get the heart rate nice and high. When sped up they can be a HIIT exercise in themselves.

TARGET MUSCLES:	TIME:
Glutes | Hamstrings | Quadriceps | Abductors and Adductors | Deltoids | Upper Trapezius | Abdominals *(for support)*	30 seconds

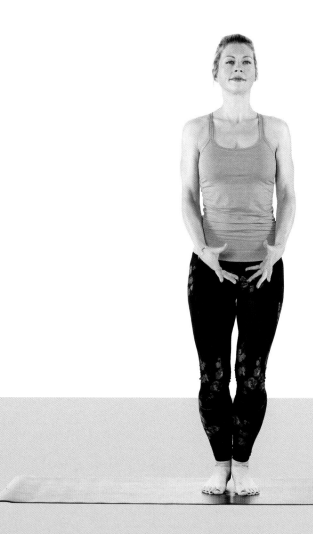

TECHNIQUE:

Start standing, feet together and arms by your sides. Jump your feet out to just wider than hip-distance apart and take the arms out to the sides and then overhead. Jump back to start.

TEACHING POINTS:

Keep the landing nice and light with soft, bouncy knees. Keep a slight bend at the elbows to prevent locking out. Keep the core engaged to prevent any leaning back. Contract the pelvic floor to help core engagement.

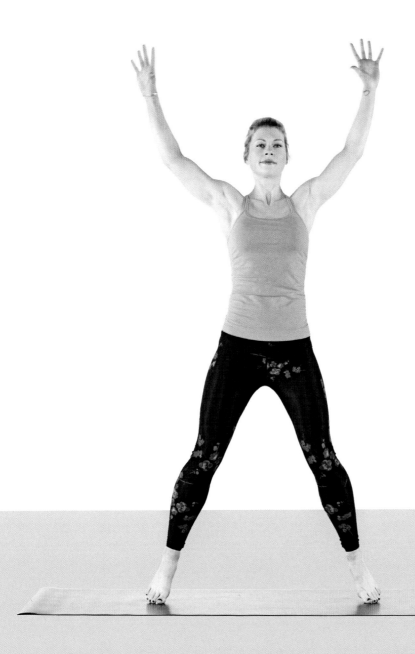

STARBURSTS

These are one of our toughest Sweat leg exercises. You'll feel the lactic acid build up in your quadriceps quite quickly but the higher you jump the harder you'll work. You may feel a little wobbly at first but that is normal.

TARGET MUSCLES:
Glutes | Quadriceps | Hamstrings | Deltoids | Abdominals *(for support)*
Calves | Hip Abductors

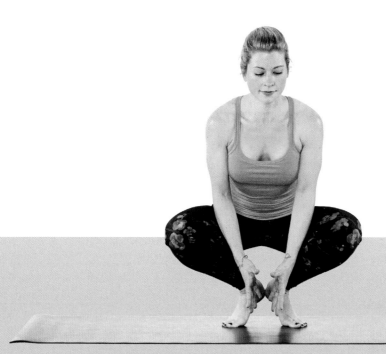

TECHNIQUE:

Start with your feet together in a V-shape, your knees bent so that they turn outwards and your fingertips reaching towards the ground. Jump up into a star shape, separating your legs and with your arms reaching out overhead. Land with your feet back together in a V-shape and bend your knees to come back to the start position.

TEACHING POINTS:

Make sure you're bending from your hips and knees and not simply hunching over to touch the floor. Keep your back nice and neutral and your core engaged. If you have tight hips, don't force yourself to actually touch the ground – go as low as is comfortable for you.

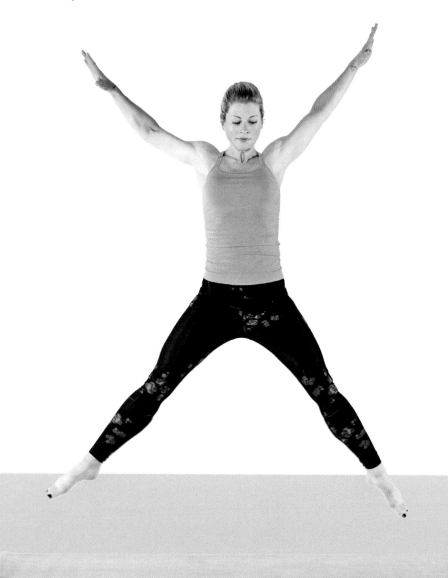

KNEE PULL

Knee pulls are a great exercise for the glutes, especially if you keep the weight in the heel of the weight-bearing foot. Imagine you are pulling down on weighted cables with your arms to create extra resistance.

TARGET MUSCLES:

Glutes | Hamstrings | Quadriceps | Back Extensors *(to maintain a neutral spine)* | Abdominals | Latissimus Dorsi | Deltoids

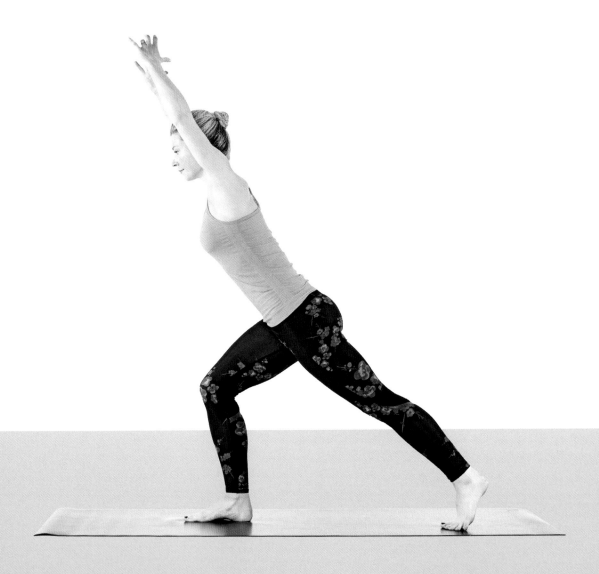

TECHNIQUE:

Start in a squat position with your weight on your right leg and your arms overhead. Pull your left knee up towards your chest and at the same time pull your arms down towards your knee. Reach your left foot back out behind you (do not touch the ground with your foot) as you take your arms back overhead. Do this for half the allotted time and swap legs half-way through.

TEACHING POINTS:

Keep your weight in your heel, maintain a neutral spine and engage your abdominals. If you feel most of the effort is in your quads, you need to try sitting back into your heel a little more. You can try adding dumb-bells to make it a little tougher.

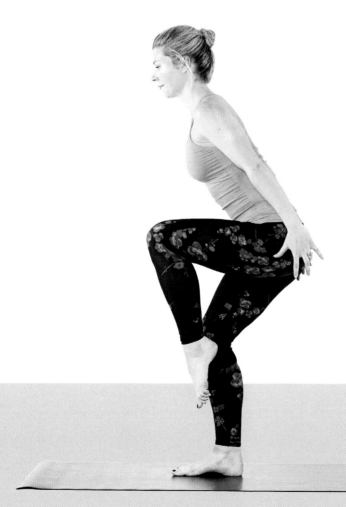

SKATERS

Skaters are fun, functional and help you visualise skiing down that black run in Switzerland. If you struggle with balance, use the non-weight-bearing leg as a support behind you but ideally stay on one leg at a time.

TARGET MUSCLES:

Glutes | Hamstrings | Quadriceps | Obliques *(to stabilise)*
Hip Abductors | Calves

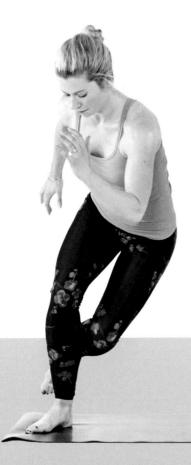

TECHNIQUE:

Start at the right-hand side of your mat with
your weight on your right leg. Jump to the
left-hand side of your mat and land on your
left leg, taking your right leg out behind you
for balance and dropping down into a squat
position. Repeat to your right.

TEACHING POINTS:

Use your second leg behind you for balance
like a monkey would use its tail. Try to cover
more distance rather than go as fast as you
can. The further you jump, the harder the
muscles will have to work. Use your arms to
aid momentum.

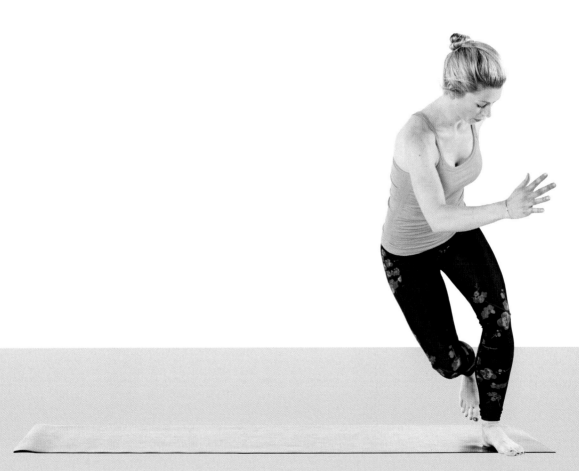

SURFERS

Surfers are great for the legs and encourage you to use plyometric (explosive) movements to allow you to turn 180 degrees. The more explosive the movement, the harder you'll work.

TARGET MUSCLES:

Glutes | Hamstrings | Quadriceps | Abdominals | Calves

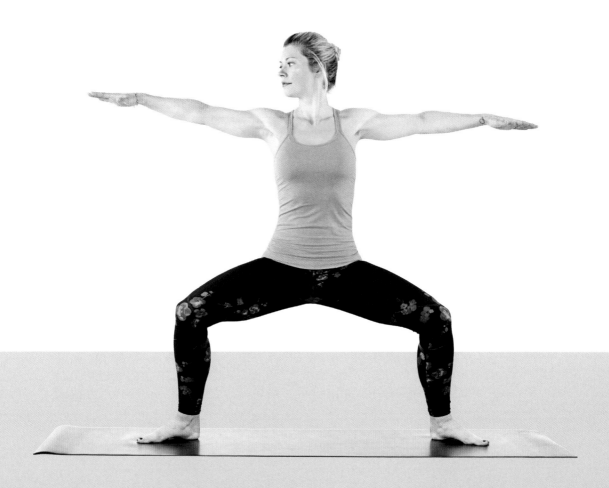

TECHNIQUE:

Imagine you are on a surfboard, feet split wider than hip-distance apart and knees bent so you are sat very low in a squat position. Your arms should be out in crucifix with you looking along your right arm. Jump up and turn 180 degrees to your right, landing in the same start position and looking along your left arm. Jump and turn 180 degrees back the way you came (to your left) and land looking along your right arm.

TEACHING POINTS:

Sit low into your squats so you require more effort to jump and manage a 180 degree turn. Keep the tailbone tucked under so you have a neutral pelvis. Bring the arms in as you turn and extend as you land.

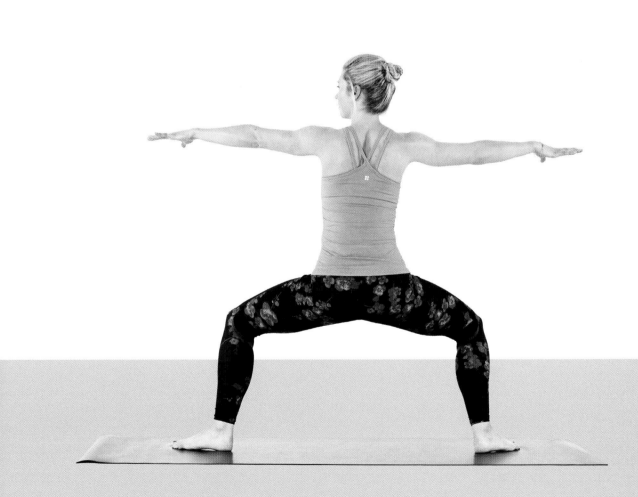

FLOOR TO CEILING

These squat jumps are great at training the fast-twitch muscles of the legs. Plyometric leg work causes the heart rate to increase quickly as it is a large muscle group.

TARGET MUSCLES:
Glutes | Hamstrings | Quadriceps | Abdominals *(for support)* | Deltoids *(to lift the arms)*

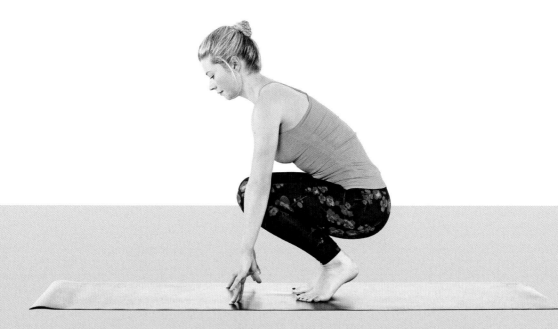

TECHNIQUE:

Stand with your feet hip-distance apart and your arms by your sides. Bend at the knees and hips into a squat and lean forwards to reach your fingers towards the floor. Make an explosive jump up to the ceiling as high as you can and reach your arms overhead as if trying to touch the ceiling above you. As soon as you land, bend at the knees and hips again and repeat.

TEACHING POINTS:

Make sure the movement is as smooth and fluid as possible. Land as softly as you can by bending the knees as soon as you touch the floor. Make sure you don't lean back as you jump up – keep a neutral pelvis.

KNEEL UPS

If you have lazy glutes, this one is great for you! I find that most people feel their glutes in this exercise, especially if they lean forwards into the move and drive their heel into the floor.

TARGET MUSCLES:

Glutes | Hamstrings | Hip Flexors | Quadriceps

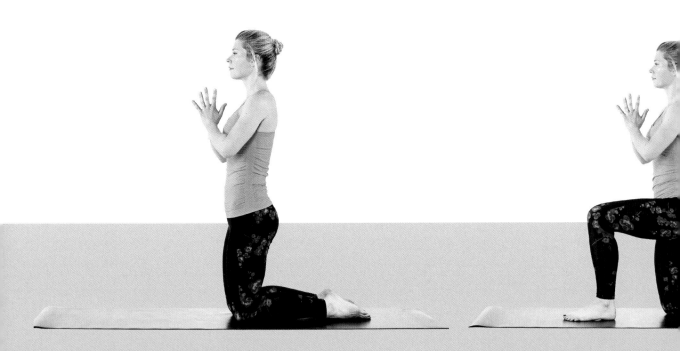

TECHNIQUE:

Start by kneeling on the floor with your hands in prayer. Step your left foot onto the floor in front of you and, using purely your left foot, push yourself up to standing and put your right foot on the floor too. Bend your left knee and come slowly down to rest your left knee back on the floor. Repeat for half the allotted time and then swap legs.

TEACHING POINTS:

Drive your weight through the heel as you stand up – this will activate the glutes. Make sure you are using your front foot to stand up. If you have dodgy knees, this is one to avoid as it can be painful.

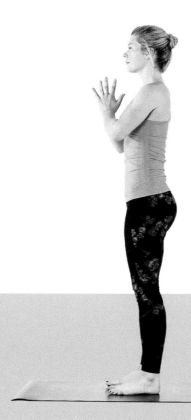

THREE-BOUNCE BURPEES

As if burpees weren't hard enough – this version is even more taxing on the quads, hamstrings and glutes, but well worth it!

TARGET MUSCLES:
Glutes | Hamstrings | Quadriceps | Abdominals
Back Stabilisers | Pectorals | Deltoids

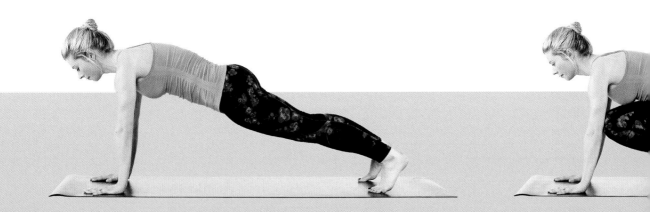

TECHNIQUE:

Start in a standing position. Bend at the knees
and place your hands down on the floor in
front of you. Jump out into a plank position
(be careful not to let the hips drop too low).
Jump your feet back to your hands and then
spring up and jump as high as you can with
your hands behind you or reaching up to the
ceiling. When you land, bend your knees down
into a squat before jumping up again (this is 1
of 3 jumps). Repeat for another 2 jumps before
placing your hands back on the floor and
jumping back out into a plank again.

TEACHING POINTS:

Try not to hunch over to reach the floor –
bend from the knees and hips. Make sure that
as you jump out into a plank your hips are in
line with the rest of the body.

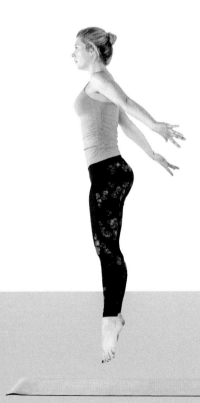

HALF BURPEES

Half burpees are a great way to practise the plank part of your burpees. Taking them slowly at first will help you assess where you are feeling the exercise (it shouldn't be in your lower back!). It's also a great challenge for the arms if you are building up to push-ups.

TARGET MUSCLES:
All the muscles of the core | Hip Flexors | Pectorals | Deltoids | Latissimus Dorsi | Quadriceps | Glutes

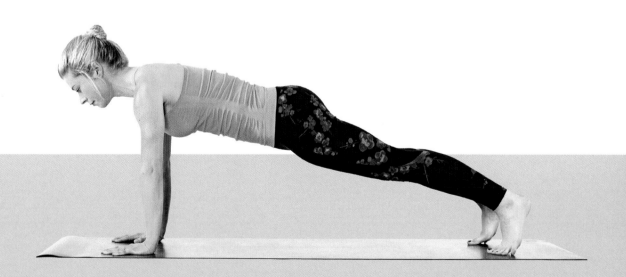

TECHNIQUE:

Start in a plank position with a neutral pelvis
and feet hip-width apart. Keeping your hands
on the ground, jump your feet up towards
your hands and land on your feet. Jump back
out into your plank and repeat.

TEACHING POINTS:

Ensure you are jumping out into a long,
neutral line. Maintain neutral scapulae,
ensuring the shoulder blades don't creep up
to the ears, and press down into the ground
to prevent winging of the scapula. Try to land
gently and smoothly.

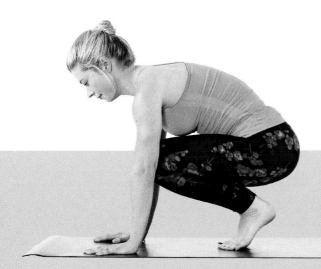

TOMBSTONES

Tombstones will never look glamourous or smooth unfortunately, but they are a great challenge and very functional (think how often you have to get yourself up to standing position each day). Using your hands is totally allowed but not using them is harder.

TARGET MUSCLES:
Abdominals | Glutes | Hamstrings | Calves | Quadriceps
Deltoids | Upper Trapezius | Hip Flexors

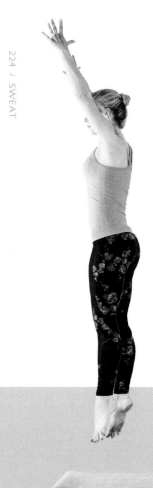

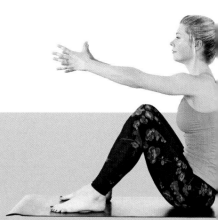

TECHNIQUE:

Start standing at one end of your mat, facing away from the mat. Jump up and reach your arms up overhead. When you land, slowly bend at the knees and lower your bum down to the floor (remember you can use your hands). Lie down carefully onto your back, straightening your legs and placing your arms overhead. From here first use your abdominals to crunch up and then your legs to help push you up to standing. Start all over again.

TEACHING POINTS:

It is better to use your hands to help you get up off the floor and/or protect you as you lower your bum back to the floor than to crash land. Try to initiate the movement of coming up from the floor using your abdominals, not your legs. When you finish the exercise and begin again with the jump, aim to jump nice and high.

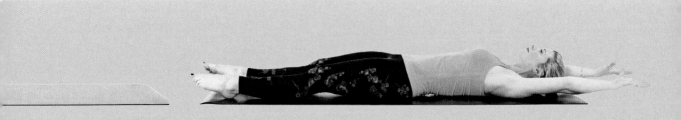

SHOULDER TAPS

Shoulder taps are a great way to challenge the obliques as they work hard to stabilise the hips and prevent them rocking from side to side. Go slow at first until you are able to maintain a neutral pelvis, then speed up.

TARGET MUSCLES:
Obliques | Pectorals | Latissimus Dorsi | Spine Extensors | Glutes

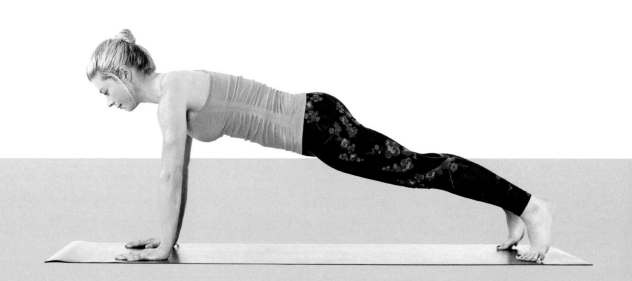

TECHNIQUE:

Start in a strong plank position, feet hip-width apart and with a neutral pelvis and scapulae. Take one hand away from the floor and tap the opposite shoulder with it. Place the hand back on the ground and pick the other hand up and tap the opposite shoulder. Repeat.

TEACHING POINTS:

Keep the hips nice and still and make sure you maintain a neutral pelvis throughout. The closer your feet are together, the harder this exercise is. Try to start slow at first, making sure you can keep technique as you pick up the pace. If it is a struggle, try lifting the hand just an inch off the floor rather than tapping the shoulder.

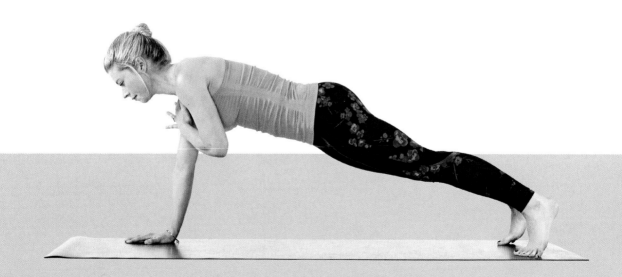

WALK THE PLANK

These are a great way to challenge core strength but is an advanced exercise, so if you have any back or shoulder issues you should avoid this.

TARGET MUSCLES:

Rectus Abdominis | Obliques | Transversus Abdominis | Deltoids | Pectorals
Latissimus Dorsi | Spine Extensors | Glutes | Hip Flexors

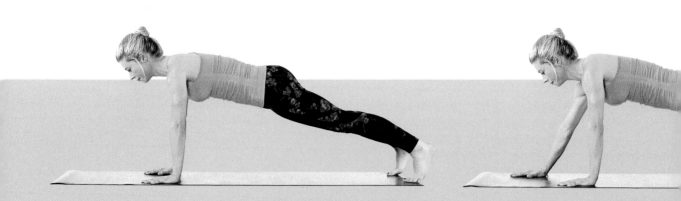

TECHNIQUE:

Start in a strong plank position, feet hip-width apart and with a neutral pelvis and scapulae. Begin to walk the hands slowly, one at a time, forwards as far as you can maintain a neutral pelvis before reversing and walking the hands back to a plank position. Repeat.

TEACHING POINTS:

You should not feel any pain during this exercise – if you do, it is not for you. Ensure there is no rocking from side to side as you walk the hands forwards and engage your core to maintain a neutral pelvis. Press into the fingertips to prevent sinking into the shoulders and engage your pelvic floor to assist the transversus abdominis.

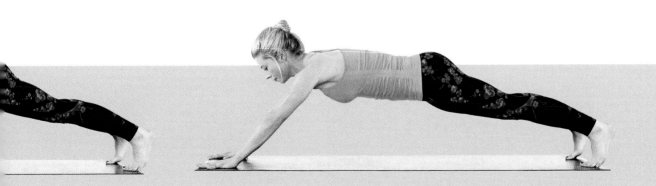

PLANK KICK-THROUGHS

These are great for engaging the obliques, challenging your balance and improving shoulder stability. Keep it slow at first and build up your speed as you progress.

TARGET MUSCLES:

Obliques | Rectus Abdominis | Transversus Abdominis | Latissimus Dorsi | Deltoids
Pectorals | Hip Abductors | Hip Adductors | Glutes | Spine | Extensors

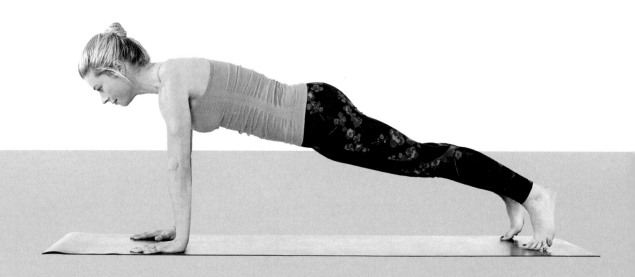

TECHNIQUE:

Start in a strong plank position, feet hip-width apart and with a neutral pelvis and scapulae. Lift your right foot off the floor and swing it under your body and between your right arm and left leg. Rotate the body to the left and lift your left hand up towards the ceiling, ending in a side plank with the right leg straight out in front of your hips, lifted away from the floor.

TEACHING POINTS:

Be careful of where you place your hand back down – make sure you are always coming back to a strong plank position in between each rep. Remember technique is key. If you are struggling to lift the leg when in your side plank, feel free to rest it on the floor and practise the full version at your own pace and without time pressures.

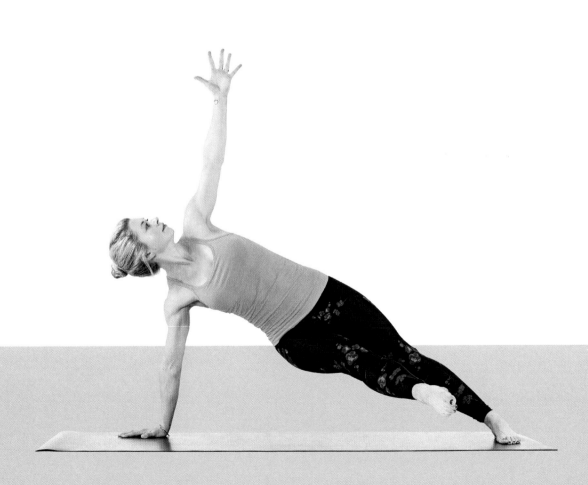

MONKEY ROPE

This exercise is great for challenging coordination (you'll have to focus on the job in hand) and for strengthening the hip flexors and core. Try to imagine you genuinely are a monkey climbing up a rope.

TARGET MUSCLES:

Hip Flexors | Rectus Abdominis | Deltoids

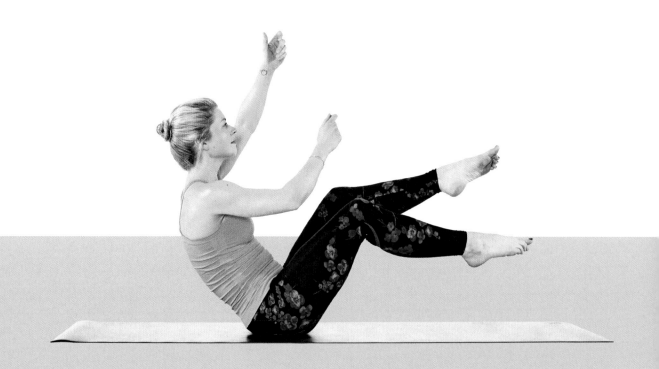

TECHNIQUE:

Start seated on your bottom with your knees bent and feet on the floor. Round your spine and lean back onto the sitting bones – your feet should now feel light and it should be easy to lift them. Reach your arms up to the ceiling and pretend you are climbing an imaginary rope using both your arms and your legs – one arm reaches up as the opposite leg reaches up.

TEACHING POINTS:

Try to keep the spine in flexion without hunching and causing tension in your neck and shoulders. This should be an exercise that challenges your stability and requires you to use your rectus abdominis to prevent you rolling backwards. Make sure to reach up high for the rope to work the deltoids and speed up as your strength improves.

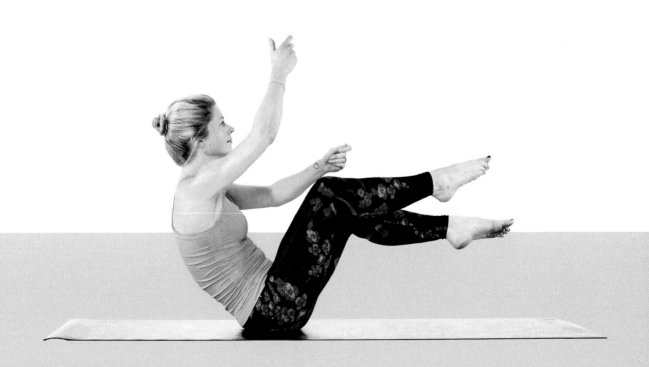

SWING PLANKS

Swing planks are a great exercise for strengthening the rotator muscles of the trunk whilst challenging shoulder stability. Keep your range of movement within your flexibility levels to ensure you don't cause tension in the lower back.

TARGET MUSCLES:

Obliques | Multifidus | Pectorals | Latissimus Dorsi | Rhomboids | Glutes

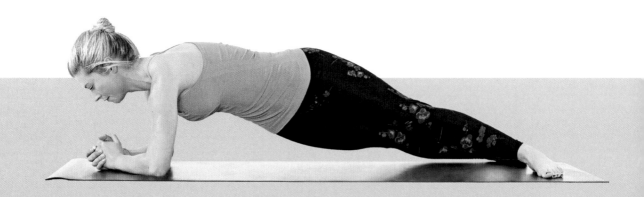

TECHNIQUE:

Start in a strong plank position, hands clasped in front of you, feet hip-width apart and with a neutral pelvis and scapulae. Rotate the hips to the right and lower the right hip towards the floor. Come back up to the start position and then rotate the left hip towards the floor. Repeat, alternating sides.

TEACHING POINTS:

Make sure you maintain a neutral pelvis to prevent any tension in the lumbar spine and keep the scapulae neutral – no sinking into your arms. You can take your feet from side to side as you rotate to make this more comfortable too.

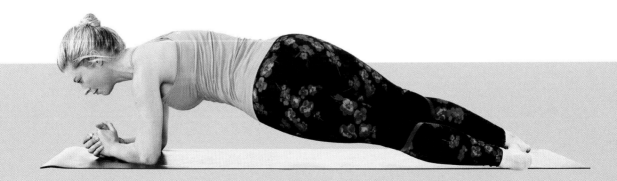

PLANK TO PIKE

This is a great exercise for the core and shoulders that also give you an effective stretch for the posterior muscles. I've always loved pikes and how they open up my shoulders after hours at my laptop.

TARGET MUSCLES:

Deltoids | Rectus Abdominis | Pectorals | Hip Flexors

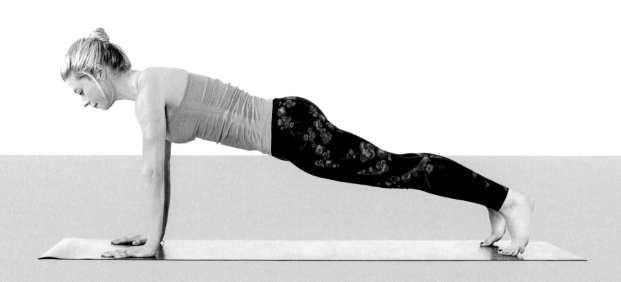

TECHNIQUE:

Start in a strong plank position, feet hip-width apart and with a neutral pelvis and scapulae. Press into your hands, draw in through the tummy and fold your body in half at the hips (you should look like a triangle with your bum in the air). Lower yourself back down into a plank and repeat.

TEACHING POINTS:

Try to use an equal amount of effort in your abdominals and arms to lift the hips. Press into your fingers and lift your heels nice and high throughout. If you have very tight hamstrings, you can always have soft knees at the top to reduce the tension.

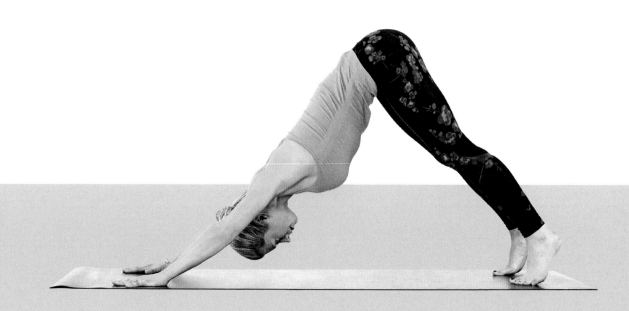

TRIANGLE PUSH-UPS

Triangle push-ups are a great way to target the pectorals. If you are kyphotic or slump at a computer all day, you would be better practising the Pilates Push-ups (page 180) instead as these focus on the triceps more.

TARGET MUSCLES:

Pectorals | Triceps | Abdominals | All muscles of the back

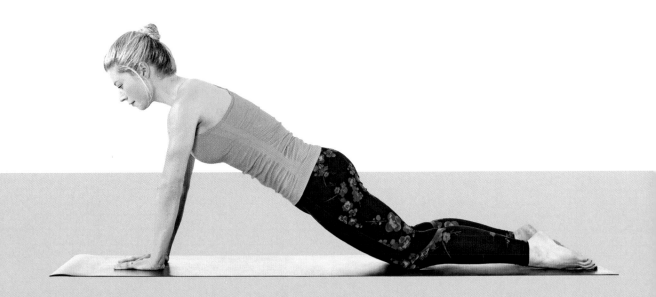

TECHNIQUE:

Start in a half plank position (or full plank if you are very strong) with your hands drawn together into a triangle shape (forefingers and thumbs touching) and flat on the floor underneath your chest, arms straight. Bend at the elbows and lower the body down towards the floor, keeping the body in a long, straight line. Straighten the arms back out, pushing yourself back to the start position. Repeat.

TEACHING POINTS:

Try to keep your scapulae in a neutral position and flat across your back (no winging). Engage the core to ensure that you maintain a neutral pelvis as you move. Only lower yourself as far as you can maintain technique, and build up your range as you get stronger.

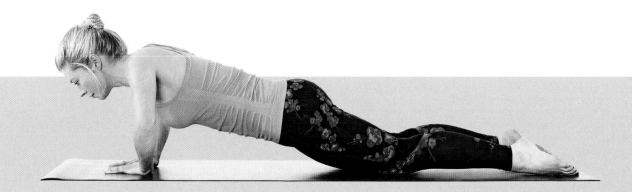

DONKEY KICKS

These are great for building arm strength and if you are learning to handstand in yoga.
They require you to put your entire weight through your arms and use your core to lift your hips.

TARGET MUSCLES:
Deltoids | Pectorals | Upper Trapezius | Abdominals |
Quadriceps | Glutes | Calves | Hip Flexors

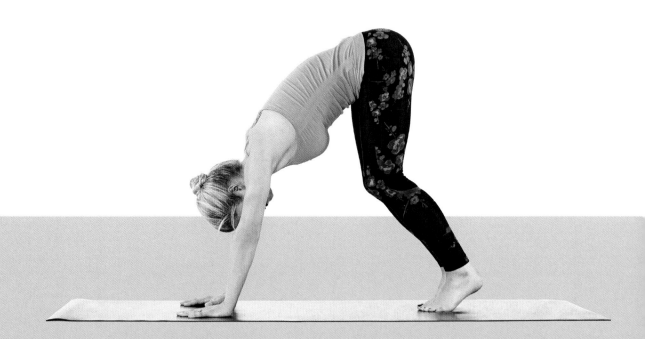

TECHNIQUE:

Start with your hands and knees on the floor, toes tucked under and scapulae neutral. Lift your knees up off the floor and take your bum into the air, leaving a slight bend in the knees (this is your start position). Press into your hands, push your feet away from the floor and lift your legs up into the air as if you are trying to kick your bum. Come down with control and bend the knees a little on landing before jumping back up into the air. Repeat.

TEACHING POINTS:

Try not to let the shoulders creep up too close to your ears. Spread your fingers wide and really grip the floor with them to encourage stability and balance. Use your core to help lift the feet high.

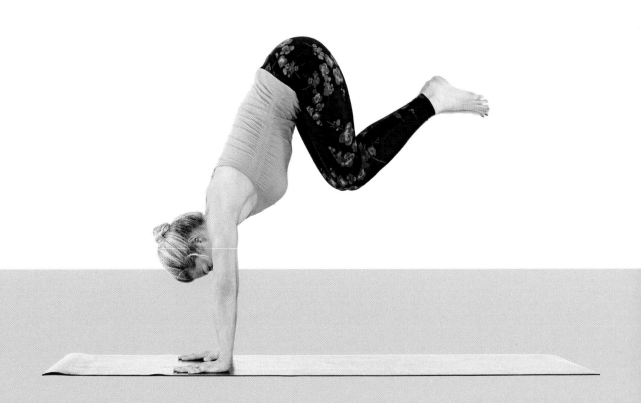

PUSH-UP TO SIDE PLANK

This movement covers a lot of bases. The side plank works the obliques and challenges the core while the push-up is great for strengthening the arms and shoulders.

TARGET MUSCLES:

Obliques | Pectorals | Deltoids | Abdominals | Glutes | Hip Abductors

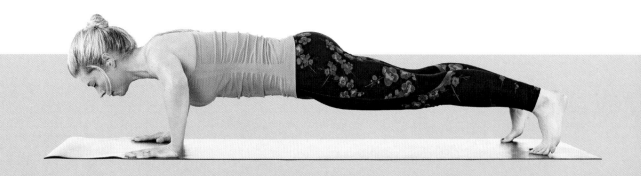

TECHNIQUE:

Start in a strong plank position, feet hip-width apart and with a neutral pelvis and scapulae. Your hands should be shoulder-width apart. Bend the elbows, drawing them back towards your hips, lowering your body down towards the ground. Straighten the arms, bringing your body back to start. Rotate the hips and flip over into a side plank, taking your top arm up to the ceiling. Rotate back to your plank start position. Repeat, alternating your side planks from side to side.

TEACHING POINTS:

Bending your elbows backwards when carrying out a push-up takes the effort away from the pecs slightly and increases the effort in the triceps. Ensure that the elbows are staying tight to the body as they bend. Make sure you maintain a neutral pelvis throughout and keep a strong diagonal line when in your side plank.

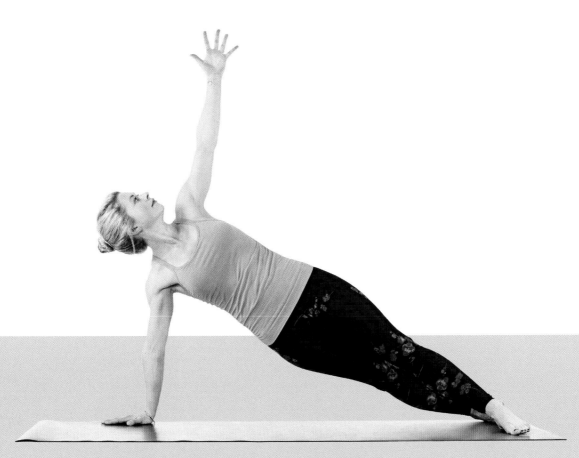

CAN CAN

This exercise is a real challenge for the arms while also encouraging oblique engagement. A half plank version is more appropriate for beginners. Whichever version you do, keep the movement slow at first.

TARGET MUSCLES:
Triceps | Rhomboids | Pectorals | Deltoids | Abdominals | Glutes | Obliques

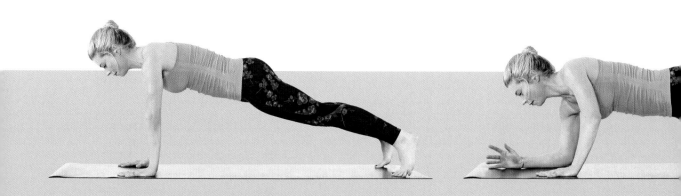

TECHNIQUE:

Start in a strong plank position, feet hip-width apart and with a neutral pelvis and scapulae. Lift your right hand off the floor and drop down slowly onto your right forearm. Then do the same with the left arm. Now put your right hand back on the floor and straighten the arm bringing your body back up before putting your left hand back on the floor too. Next time go down onto your left forearm first so you alternate each side.

TEACHING POINTS:

Try to keep the hips level as much as possible, using your obliques to stabilise. Make sure you press into the first hand to push yourself back into a plank – not the forearm left on the ground. Maintain a neutral pelvis throughout. If you are feeling the exercise in your back, please do drop the knees down and make this a half plank.

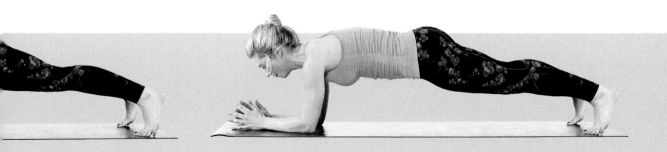

MONKEY WALK

This really works the whole body as well as the arms so is a great one for getting the heart rate lifted. Keep the knees a little soft as you walk in and out and speed up as you get stronger.

TARGET MUSCLES:
Back Extensors | Abdominals | Glutes | Pectorals | Deltoids | Upper Trapezius

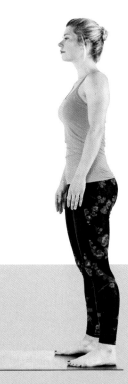

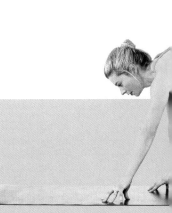

TECHNIQUE:

Start standing tall at the end of your mat, facing the mat. Roll down with control and place your hands on the ground. Walk your hands out until you are in a plank position. Walk your hands back in towards your feet and stand up one vertebra at a time until you reach the start position. Repeat.

TEACHING POINTS:

Ensure you bend your knees to take your hands down towards the floor rather than hunching over. Make sure you engage your glutes and core as you stand back up. Aim for a neutral pelvis when you're in your plank position – don't let the hips drop too low.

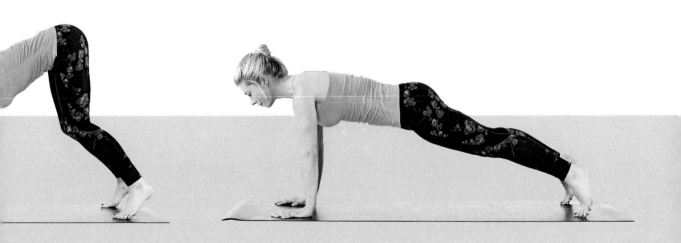

CONCLUSION

I hope this book has helped to highlight the vast reasons why exercising and eating balanced meals, rather than dieting, is the most valuable thing you can do for your health. Mindset is a powerful tool and by replacing negative thoughts regarding your body with loving and nurturing thoughts, you will make more positive decisions on a day-to-day basis. Treat your body like it is your best friend, rather than your worst enemy, and it will repay you indefinitely. You only get one body and it goes through a lot.

I want to finish by summarising my top tips and goals that I hope will set you free from the cycle of dieting and low body confidence. You deserve to love your body in its entirety – remember that the body you hate, someone else would love!

1. **Give up the diets.** They never end well. Inactivity can do more damage to your body than being overweight, so take the emphasis away from losing weight and instead focus on improving your activity levels.

2. **Love not loathe.** Exercise because you love your body, not hate it. Keep in mind all the health benefits gained from exercise and move more because you deserve to have a healthy body – not because you hate your current weight.

3. **Take a compliment.** If someone gives you a compliment, don't brush it away or deny it. Accept it and say thank you. Then write it down on a small piece of paper and put it in a jar. Whenever you need a reminder of how amazing you are, pick out one of the compliments and take it in all over again.

4. **Give out the right compliments.** Think about the message you are giving your daughter, sister, friend or colleague. We often compliment women when they have lost weight, but there are so many more worthwhile compliments to give. Tell someone how great they are at their job. Or how their company makes you so happy. This will help set other women free from the aesthetics trap.

5. **Eat with love.** Enjoy the process of sourcing, cooking and eating your food. Cook for others and accept food from them. See food as a way of sharing experiences and enjoyment, not counting calories and restricting yourself.

6. **Do not underestimate the power of your mental health.** What we think shapes how we behave. If you feel lonely, depressed, anxious or overwhelmed, please seek help. Mental health issues are not rare and you will not be alone. There is support out there. Please do not try to fix your unhappiness by losing weight.

I wish you all the best on your journey. You are amazing and deserve to be healthy, happy and strong. You can learn to love yourself – start now!

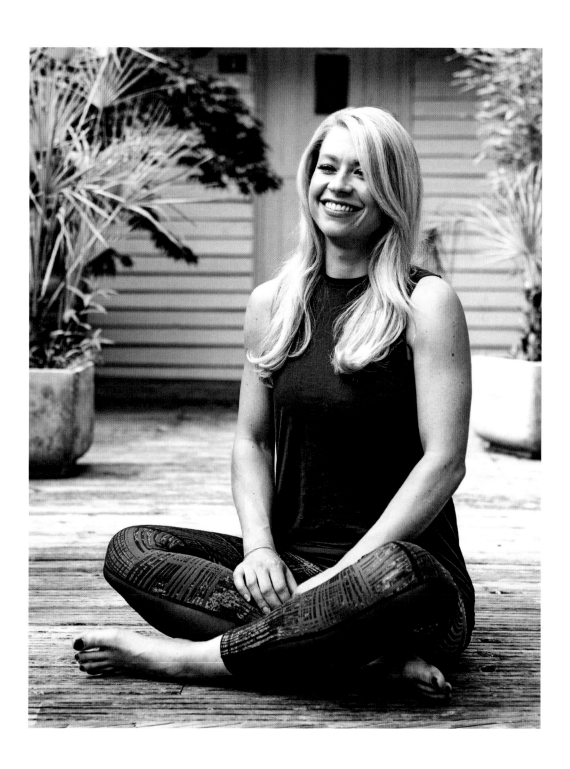

REFERENCES

1. Tim Spector, The Diet Myth: The Real Science Behind What We Eat (London: Weidenfeld & Nicolson, 2015).

2. Marie Ng, Tom Fleming, Margaret Robinson, et al., 'Global, regional, and national prevalence of overweight and obesity in children and adults during 1980–2013: A systematic analysis for the Global Burden of Disease Study 2013', The Lancet, 2014, Vol. 384 (No. 9945), 766–81.

3. T. Mann, A. J. Tomiyama, E. Westling, A.-M. Lew, B. Samuels and J. Chatman, 'Medicare's search for effective obesity treatments: Diets are not the answer', American Psychologist, 2007, Vol. 62, 220–33.

4. N. Townsend, K. Wickramasinghe, J. Williams, P. Bhatnagar and M. Rayner, National Activity Statistics 2015 (London: British Heart Foundation, 2015).

5. Anna Kessel, Eat Sweat Play: How Sport Can Change Our Lives (London: Macmillan, 2016).

6. Girlguiding, Girls' Attitudes Survey (Girlguiding, 2016), https://www.girlguiding.org.uk/globalassets/docs-and-resources/research-and-campaigns/girls-attitudes-survey-2016.pdf.

7. A. J. Swerdlow, R. Peto and R. Doll, 'Epidemiology of cancer', in Oxford Textbook of Medicine, edited by D. A. Warrell, T. M. Cox and J. D. Firth, 299–332 (Oxford: Oxford University Press, 2010).

8. Ulf Ekelund et al., 'Physical activity and all-cause mortality across levels of overall and abdominal adiposity in European men and women: The European Prospective Investigation into Cancer and Nutrition Study (EPIC)', American Journal of Clinical Nutrition, 2015, Vol. 101 (No. 3), 613–21.

9. Tracy L. Tylka, Rachel A. Annunziato, Deb Burgard, et al., 'The weight-inclusive versus weight-normative approach to health: Evaluating the evidence for prioritizing well-being over weight loss', Journal of Obesity, 2014, Vol. 2014, Art. 983495.

10. Food Standards Agency, The Eatwell Guide (2016), https://www.food.gov.uk/northern-ireland/nutritionni/eatwell-guide.

11. Public Health England, Patterns and Trends in Adult Diets, http://webarchive.nationalarchives.gov.uk/20160805121933/http://noo.org.uk/securefiles/160805_1340//Adult-dietfactsheetDec2015.pdf

12. American Dietetic Association and Dietitians of Canada, 'Position of the American Dietetic Association and Dietitians of Canada: Vegetarian diets', Journal of the American Dietetic Association, 2003, Vol. 103, 748–65.

13. Public Health England, Health Survey for England – 2014 (Leeds: Health and Social Care Information Centre, 2015).

14. H. M. Orpana, J.-M. Berthelot, M. S. Kaplan, et al., 'BMI and mortality: Results from a national longitudinal study of Canadian adults', Obesity, 2010, Vol. 18, 214–18.

15. M. S. Kaplan, N. Huguet, J. T. Newsom, B. H. McFarland and J. Lindsay, 'Prevalence and correlates of overweight and obesity among older adults: Findings from the Canadian National Population Health Survey', Journals of Gerontology A: Biological Sciences and Medical Sciences, 2003, Vol. 58, 1018–30.

16. B. Khoury, M. Sharma, S. E. Rush and C. Fournier, 'Mindfulness-based stress reduction for healthy individuals: A meta-analysis', Journal of Psychosomatic Research, 2015, Vol. 78 (No. 6), 519–28.

17. L. B. Andersen, P. Schnohr, M. Schroll and H. O. Hein, 'All-cause mortality associated with physical activity during leisure time, work, sports, and cycling to work', Archives of Internal Medicine, 2000, Vol. 160 (No. 11), 1621–28.

18. Roald Bahr and Ole M. Sejersted, 'Effect of intensity of exercise on excess postexercise O2 consumption', Metabolism, 1991, Vol. 40 (No. 8), 836–41.

19. M. Heydari, J. Freund and S. H. Boutcher, 'The effect of high-intensity intermittent exercise on body composition of overweight young males', Journal of Obesity, 2012, Vol. 2012, Art. 480467.

20. Stephen H. Boutcher, 'High-intensity intermittent exercise and fat loss', Journal of Obesity, 2011, Vol. 2011, Art. 868305.

21. J. L. Kuk, P. T. Katzmarzyk, M. Z. Nichaman, T. S. Church, S. N. Blair and R. Ross, 'Visceral fat is an independent predictor of all-cause mortality in men', Obesity, 2006, Vol. 14 (No. 2), 336–41.

22. I. Tabata, K. Nishimura, M. Kouzaki et al., 'Effects of moderate-intensity endurance and high-intensity intermittent training on anaerobic capacity and VO(2max)', Medicine and Science in Sports and Exercise, 1996, Vol. 28 (No. 10), 1327–30.

23. T. A. Astorino, R. P. Allen, D. W. Roberson and M. Jurancich, 'Effect of high-intensity interval training on cardiovascular function, VO2max, and muscular force', Journal of Strength and Conditioning Research, 2012, Vol. 26 (No. 1), 138–45.

24. P. Boudou, E. Sobngwi, F. Mauvais-Jarvis, P. Vexiau and J.-F. Gautier, 'Absence of exercise-induced variations in adiponectin levels despite decreased abdominal adiposity and improved insulin sensitivity in type 2 diabetic men', European Journal of Endocrinology, 2003, Vol. 149 (No. 5), 421–24.

25. E. G. Trapp, D. J. Chisholm, J. Freund and S. H. Boutcher, 'The effects of high-intensity intermittent exercise training on fat loss and fasting insulin levels of young women', International Journal of Obesity, 2008, Vol. 32 (No. 4), 684–91.

26. Angelo Tremblay, Jean-Aimé Simoneau and Claude Bouchard, 'Impact of exercise intensity on body fatness and skeletal muscle metabolism', Metabolism, 1994, Vol. 43 (No. 7), 814–18.

INDEX

A

adductors 121, 122
ADP (adenosine diphosphate) 190, 191
aerobic respiration 190–1
agonists 120
alcohol 29
amino acids 24–6
anaerobic respiration 190–1
anatomy 118–27
  joints 118–20
  muscles 120–6
  spine 127
  animal antibiotics 23–4
  antagonists 120
ATP (adenosine triphosphate) 190, 191, 192

B

beta-carotene 20
bicep curls 120
biceps 121, 124
blood flow 191
blood pressure 20
blood sugar levels 22, 34, 195
BMI (body mass index) 16, 30–1
body fat 34–5, 194
breastfeeding 132
breathing
  effect of exercise on 186
  Pilates breath patterns 136

C

calcium 22, 23, 118
calves 121, 123
carbohydrates 21–3, 33
cartilage 118
cervical spine 127
cholesterol 32
circulation 187–8
coccyx spine 127
complex sugars 22

computer work 129, 132
cortisol 35
crucifix 117

D

daily activities 131–4
  breastfeeding 132
  carrying heavy weights 133
  computer work 129, 132
  leaning over 129, 132–3
  sitting 126, 131–2
  sitting cross-legged 133
dairy 23–4
dehydration 29
deltoids 121, 125
depression 37
diaphragm muscles 121, 125
dieting, effects of 17–18
DOMS (delayed-onset muscle soreness) 26
dopamine 27

E

eating disorders 18
emotional eating 27
EPOC (excess post-exercise oxygen consumption) 192
erector spinae 121, 123
essential fatty acids 32
exercises
  effects of 185–92, 194–5
  STRENGTHEN
    CORE
      criss cross 158–9
      hip twist 168–9
      hundreds 154–5
      kyphosis corrector 166–7
      mermaid plank 162–3
      scissors 160–1
      single-leg stretch 156–7
      swimming 164–5
    LOWER BODY

arabesque deadlift 140–1
elevated clam 144–5
scooter 146–7
ship 142–3
side-lying leg raise 148–9
single-leg lift 150–1
single-leg squat 152–3
UPPER BODY
cactus 172–3
dumb waiter 176–7
incline push-up 178–9
leg pull prep 174–5
Pilates push-up 180–1
single-arm push up 170–1
SWEAT
CORE
monkey rope 232–3
plank kick-throughs 230–1
shoulder taps 226–7
swing planks 234–5
three-bounce burpees 222–3
tombstones 224–5
walk the plank 228–9
LOWER BODY
floor to ceiling 216–17
half burpees 220–1
knee pulls 210–11
kneel ups 218–19
skaters 212–13
starbursts 208–9
surfers 214–15
UPPER BODY
can can 244–5
donkey kicks 240–1
monkey walk 246–7
plank to pike 236–7
push-up to side plank 242–3
triangle push-ups 238–9
WARM-UPS
high knees 204–5
jumping jacks 206–7
squat rotations 202–3
exertion scale 196

F
fat, dietary 24, 27, 32–3
fibre 20
flat back posture 128, 130
folate 20
fructose 22
fruit 20–1

G
galactose 22, 23
gaseous exchange 186
ghrelin 17
glucose 22, 23, 190, 195
gluteals 121, 122
glycogen 22
government guidelines 18–30
    carbohydrates 21–3
    dairy 23–4
    fat 27
    hydration 29
    protein 22, 24–6
    sugar 27–9
    vegetables/fruit 20–1

H
hamstrings 121, 122
HDLs (high-density lipoproteins) 33
head placement 138
heart rate 188, 196
heart rate monitors 196
heavy objects, carrying 133
HIIT (high-intensity interval training) 184, 192, 194–6, 198
hip flexors 121, 123
homeostasis 186, 191, 192
hormones 17, 26, 27, 34, 35, 38, 186, 195
hydration 29

I
imprint 117, 137
insulin sensitivity 195
involuntary muscles 120, 188

iron 20, 22

J
joints 118–20

K
knee joints 119
kyphosis 129
kyphotic-lordotic posture 128, 129, 132

L
lactic acid 190–1, 192, 198
lactose 23
lactose intolerance 23
latissimus dorsi 121, 124
LDLs (low-density lipoproteins) 32, 33
leaning over 129, 132–3
ligaments 118
lipoproteins 32–3
lordosis 129–30
lumbar spine 127
lycopene 20

M
maximum heart rate 196
mindful eating 38–9
mindfulness 35, 37–9
minerals 20, 22, 23, 118
monounsaturated fats 33
multifidus 121, 124
muscle imbalances 126, 131–5
    prevention of 134–5
muscles 120–6

N
neck flexors 121, 125
neutral pelvis 117, 136–7

O
obesity 6, 30–1
obliques 121, 123
omega 3 fats 26, 33
omega 6 fats 33
organic products 24
over-stretching 119

overweight 6, 16

P
pectorals 121, 124
pelvic floor 121, 122
pelvic placement 136–7
    imprint 117, 137
    neutral pelvis 117, 136–7
phytochemicals 20
Pilates
    history of 114–15
    principles 135–8
Pilates, Joseph Hubertus 114–15
polyunsaturated fats 33
posture types 128–31
    flat back 128, 130
    kyphotic–lordotic 128, 129, 132
    sway back 128, 130–1
potassium 20
protein 22, 24–6, 33

Q
quadriceps 121, 123

R
recipes
    BREAKFAST
    baked black beans, coriander guacamole and
        poached eggs 46–7
    banana and oat energy bars 45
    corn and lime fritters 50
    orange and sea salt granola 52
    savoury thyme porridge 49
    smoked salmon, egg and turmeric muffins 55
    vanilla multigrain porridge 48
    DESSERT
    apple, apricot and thyme crumble 104
    cacao, mint and hazelnut pots 108
    chocolatier's hot chocolate 101
    praline nice-cream 105
    roast figs with orange, honey and pistachios
        110
    rosemary and chocolate banana bread 102
    spiced poached plums 106
    DINNER

chilli and sesame tuna poke bowl 76
Indian spiced oat fried chicken with chilli
    and coriander corn 69
roast chicken 71
salmon, lemongrass and ginger patties 78
speltsotto 74
squash and leek gratin 72
steak and black bean burritos with coriander
    guacamole 80–1
wholewheat spaghetti 79
ENTERTAINING
beetroot, fennel, thyme and goats' cheese
    tart 88
cashew and oat pancakes with peaches,
    orange yoghurt and bacon 84
lamb, chickpea and apricot tagine 89
lentil dal, spiced roast cauliflower and mint
    yoghurt 86–7
roast chicken thighs 90
squash and rosemary carbonara 83
LUNCH
chicken stew 59
chickpea and coriander falafel wraps with
    sweet chilli sauce 64–5
chorizo, butterbean, spelt and kale broth 57
fig, mozzarella and candied walnut salad 61
nourish bowl 62
pea, edamame and mint frittata 66
Thai slaw salad 60
SIDES
apricot, mint and pistachio quinoa 98
aubergine and harissa hummus 93
beetroot, orange and poppy seed salad 99
green beans with crispy shallots, pine nuts
    and garlic 94
soy, sesame and honey-glazed carrots 95
spicy Thai fried aubergine 94
rectus abdominis 121, 124
rhomboids 121, 125
ribcage placement 137

S
sacral spine 127
saturated fats 32, 33
scapula placement 137–8

seasonal eating 40
seasonal produce list 41
sedentary life-style 126, 131–2, 133
simple sugars 22
sleep 35
spine 127
starchy foods 21–3, 33
stress 35
stroke volume 188
subcutaneous fat 34, 194
sugar 22, 23, 34, 27–9
sway back posture 128, 130–1
sweat workouts 198–200
sweating 29, 191

T
tabletop 117
tendons 118
testosterone 26
thoracic spine 127
transversus abdominis 121, 124
trapezius 121, 125
triceps 121, 124

U
unsaturated fats 32, 33

V
vegan choices/practices 23, 26
vegetables 20–1
visceral fat 34–5, 194
vitamins 20
    fat-soluble 32
    vitamin A 20
    vitamin B complex 20, 21
    vitamin C 20
VO2 max 195

W
warm-ups 199, 200, 202–7
water 29

ACKNOWLEDGEMENTS

Firstly, I would like to thank Jillian, my editor, for realising I had an important message to share, and for believing in me when I would never have dreamed I would get to write my own book. The team at Little, Brown have been amazing and I will forever be grateful to them for this opportunity.

I would like to also thank my loyal clients at PilatesPT who have helped shape The Model Method, given advice and reassurance, and have always taken a passionate interest in this book and have supported me throughout the last seven years. You make all the 4.30am alarms worthwhile.

I'd like to thank Laura Thomas, PhD. for helping me ensure this book does not further muddy the nutrition waters and for her patience throughout my recipe testing.

I want to thank my ever-patient husband Stuart who has supported me through the rollercoaster of emotions that come with writing a book. He has kept our fridge stocked with wine, my tummy full and has been an important shoulder to cry on. He's a pretty amazing business partner too.

I would also like to thank my dad for passing on his competitive genes and work ethic – these traits have led me to this career. And similarly, to my brother for always having my back. Finally, I'd like to thank my mum who taught me I can do anything a man can do. You have supported me throughout this journey, despite thinking I'm mad, and are my absolute rock.